## Routledge Focus on Mental Health

Routledge Focus on Mental Health presents short books on current topics, linking in with cutting-edge research and practice.

**Efficient Therapy for Specific Client Problems**
Making the Most of Every Client Session
*Windy Dryden*

**The Mind of Complex Numbers and the Subject in Analyses**
*Raul Moncayo*

**Being a Crisis Chaplain**
Delivering Help and Healing in Critical Scenarios
*Sidney Dekker and Lance Mergard*

**A Critical Examination of Irvin D. Yalom's Single Session Consultations**
It Is the Relationship That Heals
*Windy Dryden*

**The Power of Being a Subject**
Transcending Human Mechanics with Critical Thinking, Honesty, Patience, and Bravery
*Matthew H. Bowker*

**The Knowledge of the Psychoanalyst**
*Raul Moncayo*

For more information about this series, please visit: www.routledge.com/Routledge-Focus-on-Mental-Health/book-series/RFMH

# The Knowledge of the Psychoanal

*The Knowledge of the Psychoanalyst* documents Raul Moncayo's pr analysis over a period of twenty-five years.

Exploring different aspects of knowledge in the work of Fr Lacan, Moncayo considers themes including not-knowing as op non-knowing, truth, and ignorance. The book considers unconscio $S_1$ signifiers, understandings of history as both linear and circu the different levels of mind in Mahayana Buddhism and psycho The book also presents cases of obsessional neurosis and hyster Lacanian sense. The book concludes with Moncayo's own inter of Lacan's theory, in the same way that Lacan had his own inter of Freud.

*The Knowledge of the Psychoanalyst* will be of great interest to analysts in practice and in training, and academics and scholars of theory.

**Raul Moncayo** was born in Chile and first trained as a psychoa Buenos Aires, Argentina. He obtained his PhD in social-clinical ps at the Wright Institute in Berkeley and trained as an analyst at the School of Psychoanalysis, which he also helped found. He is the of the Chinese American Center for Freudian and Lacanian Ana Research.

# The Knowledge of the Psychoanalyst

Raul Moncayo

Routledge
Taylor & Francis Group
LONDON AND NEW YORK

First published 2025
by Routledge
4 Park Square, Milton Park, Abingdon, Oxon OX14 4RN

and by Routledge
605 Third Avenue, New York, NY 10158

*Routledge is an imprint of the Taylor & Francis Group, an informa business*



*British Library Cataloguing-in-Publication Data*
A catalogue record for this book is available from the British Library

ISBN: 9781041111832 (hbk)
ISBN: 9781041111849 (pbk)
ISBN: 9781003658702 (ebk)

DOI: 10.4324/9781003658702

Typeset in Times New Roman
by KnowledgeWorks Global Ltd.

# Contents

# 1 The Knowledge of the Psychoanalyst

*Raul Moncayo and Carlos Jimenez*

*Seminar XIX* follows *Seminar XVIII* (*On a Discourse That Might Not Be a Semblance*) and is the seminar before *Seminar XX*, where Lacan introduces his formulas of sexuation. *Seminar XIX* is then followed by *Seminar XIXa*, which links the former to *Seminar XX*.

In *Seminar XIXa*, *The Knowledge of the Psychoanalyst*, Lacan ([1971–72] n.d.) talks about the professional knowledge that psychiatric interns gain in their training. Here he links knowledge to ignorance, and he relates this to how in Buddhism ignorance is considered a form of passion.

In Buddhism (Vasubhandu, 1984), ignorance is a passion because ignorance is the root cause of suffering that leads to clinging and craving. It is deluded perceptions that fuel negative emotions. We also treat reality as it existed outside our mind and not as a product of mind.

Then why do humans desire not to know? There are things that humans would rather forget and repress. But there are things that cannot be remembered because they were repressed from the beginning by the system of language. The Symbolic represses the Real so that the Real in this sense is forgotten as something impossible, or worse, as the title of *Seminar XIX*.

The mode of not-knowing or non-knowing is not of the order of repression (*Verdrängung*) but of what Freud refers to as primal repression (*Urverdrängung*). However, we argue that there are two forms of primal or primary repression, whichever we choose to call them. Freud's primary repression is a fundamental operation of an anti-cathexis in the determination of psychic life.

There is an aspect of true forgetting that supports the side of truth that remains in the Real. "In every entry of being into its habitation in words, there's a margin of forgetting, a *lethe* complementary to every a*letheia*" (Lacan, 1953–54, p. 192). This originary form of repression Moncayo (2021) has theorized as a second type of primary repression linked to the true hole of Lacan's *Seminar XXIII*: "And it is this hole that I am aiming at…that I recognize in the *Uverdrangung* itself" (9.12.75. II XVI).

This form of unconscious mind is beyond thinking. For an infant this is an experience of the world and the good breast, which is good but beyond

DOI: 10.4324/9781003658702-1

representation. The child cannot symbolize or put into words their own experience. This is Lacan's last theory of the knowledge of the psychoanalyst. This knowledge is what operates in psychoanalytic treatment. This theory developed after developing the theory of the transference as the Subject Supposed to Know (S.s.S.).

There are two levels of thinking—conscious and unconscious—and there is a form of experiential mind that is beyond thinking. What does non-thinking mean in analysis? The analysand does not think, but free associates. In addition, speech is punctuated by the silence of the analyst as a background for true speech in the analysand.

There are two types of primary repression: the one described by Freud in the metapsychological papers, and the one described by Lacan.

There are also two forms of passion for ignorance. This passion consists of two modes of negation and negativity specific to psychoanalytic experience. The first passion to repress is the cathectic force of the *Verdrängung,* and the other the anti-cathectic force of Freud's *Urverdrängung.* The anti-cathectic force of primary repression applies only to Freud's concept. This is not a passion in the sense of the sexual drive, but a passion to repress that interferes with the rule to undo the repression in analysis.

If ignorance is a passion, it is because it concerns the operation of what psychoanalysis refers to as the force of repression that the analyst is no less spared than the analysand, despite analysis being guided by the therapeutic principle of undoing repression.

Ambiguously, the analyst has to let go of the position of knowledge, but at the same time the position of knowledge is necessary for the development of the positive transference. The analyst has to represent a semblance of knowledge but also must not cling to the Subject Supposed to Know position. Not letting go of this position leads to the analyst not wanting to know anything about their ignorance. The analyst repudiates what they ignore, he rejects it, says Lacan, repression being the English translation of the *Verdrängung*, because the analyst "wants to know nothing about it" (Lacan, [1971–72] 2018, p. 14).

What kind of knowledge can be accessed only by beginning with the assumption of ignorance not as a deficit but as what is essentially linked to knowledge by making ignorance itself the basis for an established knowledge? Lacan brings the famous reference of doctoral ignorance (*docte ignorantia*) of medieval theologian Nicholas de Cusa by which the more you know that you are unknowing, the more learned you will be. But ignorance is more than superstition or lack of knowledge in the sense of data or information. You can know a lot of facts in the form of data but remain ignorant in the sense of the Buddhist ignorance (*Avidyā*). The entire internet and AI are ignorant in this sense. The metaverse is not a higher cloud of knowledge or the *topos Uranus*, the world of ideas; it is rather the world of karma and Buddhist ignorance. The metaverse or AI cannot generate new knowledge like humans do.

There's a difference between information as ignorance (*Avidyā*) and ignorance as knowledge with which one begins (*docte ignorantia*), and then there is a difference between knowledge and truth.

Truth is the experience of non-knowledge in which the One reveals itself and makes Being and non-being. Doctoral ignorance is not a lack of knowledge or silence as such, but a non-knowledge. This is what Wittgenstein (2002) discovered in two ways, first by his own assumption of the doctrine of doctoral ignorance, when he famously states in the *Tractatus Logico-Philosophicus* that "What we cannot speak about we must pass over in silence" (Wittgenstein, 1922, Proposition 7). However, Wittgenstein does not derive new forms of knowing from his silence, and silence here is not in the position of truth as in psychoanalysis.

Wittgenstein does not espouse silence as such but considers the necessity of falling silent as an entrance into the encounter with ignorance rather than non-knowledge, which he does not realize. Indeed, Wittgenstein states only two sections prior in the *Tractatus* that "There are, indeed, things that cannot be put into words. They make themselves manifest. They are what is mystical" (2002, Proposition 6.522). Wittgenstein falls silent on the thing-in-itself, but he perceives how things make themselves manifest.

In our thesis, things make themselves manifest without the thinking or the speaking of the subject, and silence becomes the form of the encounter with the Real object as the experience of non-knowledge that would be the mystical, poetic, or ineffable of the One. The subject is also included in things in this case.

How is non-knowledge different from not-knowing or ignorance in the sense of *Avidyā*? Wittgenstein answers this question in his later work, *Philosophical Investigations* (1958), where he reconsiders the place of the inexpressible (the Real) in language. Where in the *Tractatus* language functions to produce knowledge that captures or represent 'objective' facts of the world as information or data (ignorance as *Avidyā*), the *Investigations* develops a theory of language of what Wittgenstein calls 'language games' (1958, Proposition 23).

Language games consider the ways in which words contain a 'multiplicity' within them that depends on the specific context in which a word is used and how it functions within a text (Proposition 24), as metaphor and metonymy, according to Lacanian theory. In this sense, what Wittgenstein calls the mystical is not beyond language but is contained within forms of multiplicity that Wittgenstein calls 'language games'. However, this move of the game reduces the Real to language once again, although in this case it could be argued that language games involve the poetic function.

In the silence of non-knowing prescribed by the *Tractatus*, the mind is open, and one has no expectations or prejudices, while in not-knowing one simply ignores the ineffable things that "make themselves manifest" as the mystical (Proposition 6.522). Doctoral silence is the form of ignorance that is bliss. The form of experience of the truth as non-thinking, or beyond thinking, does not exist in the $S_2$ of the discourse of the analyst in Lacan's theory.

As non-knowledge, it is not simply that one does not know but that non-knowledge cannot be known as datum, fact, or information. There nevertheless is a use and function of language in Wittgenstein's theory of language games that entails that there is no 'objective' fact that remains self-same across time; rather, the words we use to describe the objective miss the ineffable and do not exhaust all possible field of meanings that an event or object assumes. Because words miss the ineffable, they are always trying to represent it by displacing unto new meaning. This is where the outside meaning operates within meaning, in an imaginary way.

In psychoanalysis, interpretation is the process by which the analyst, through verbal communication, offers insights—a tracing into the unconscious signification of a patient's thoughts, feelings, or actions—aiming to help the analysand gain awareness and understand unconscious significations. This is the classical definition of interpretation, but for Lacan ([1968–1969] 2023) an interpretation is somewhere between a citation and an enigma. Citation is a citation of what the analysand said. But the repetition, together with the tone of voice of the analyst, invokes an enigma.

The analyst's interpretation does not bring the analysand only to a place of understanding the facts of their repressed unconscious but also into contact with the mystical and ineffable contained within the signifier. Citation evokes enigmatic affects and signifiers. In addition, the analyst needs to have a sense of right timing and that the analysand is ready and able to receive the interpretation, whether consciously or unconsciously.

Enigmatic affects manifest the Real unconscious that is also present in analysis and contributes to its therapeutic value. The multiplicity of meanings generated through the effects of the signifier, although symbolic, remains within the displacements of the signifier that miss the Real. Here, the more you say, the less you truly speak.

The concept of interpretation is linked at first to the concept of information related to anamnesis, to memory, and to the history of the symptom. However, anamnestic information is not knowledge, and knowledge is not unconscious knowing, and information is not interpretation.

Interpretation is the knowledge specific to the analyst, which is derived from the poetic function of language and which enables the writing of desire in analysis. In other words, it is not psychiatric diagnosis or the laws of semiology or that are consequential in analytic interpretation but rather the very operation of interpretation that functions to generate a form of poetic discourse.

What does Lacan mean by the use of the word 'semiology' rather than 'linguistics'? Semiology is broader than linguistics and includes the use of signs in nature. In contrast to Lacan, we argue that this is the natural language, while language is cultural more than natural. It is different to say that the unconscious is structured by semiology rather than language. The idea that language is structured by semiology would agree with Freud, Jung, and Peirce.

If the unconscious is structured like a language, it means that the unconscious is ordered rather than merely a chaotic primary process. Freud believed that the unconscious was organized not by language but by contradictory images and the secondary revision provided by the dreamwork. In one sense, language is unconscious in a descriptive sense (like the preconscious); on the other hand, the unconscious can be more than linguistic. Only when Lacan invented the concept of *lalangue* and associations by homophony did the unconscious acquire its own structure, however weak. Language itself is constituted by a system of differences. But difference does not mean inconsistency; it simply means that one has to find the meaning of words by using other words.

Now, how is the symptom produced? Freud said a symptom is a substitute, and thus subject to the laws of metaphor and metonymy. Language, metaphor, and metonymy function as a system of differences as well, but metaphor and metonymy are not symptoms. A symptom is like a slip of the tongue coming from the unconscious, repetitive thoughts, or a feeling of anxiety or depression.

How is this related to what Lacan calls the disjunction between the subject and the verb? It is the subject that speaks under the semblance or mask of the ego. The word 'I' represents the subject not the ego. There is something else speaking inside the subject that is structured as a language, and this is not the ego.

In a sentence, the subject is the person, place, or thing performing the action. The verb is the action itself; therefore, the relationship between a subject and a verb is that the verb must agree with the subject in number (singular or plural) and sometimes person (first, second, or third)—meaning that if the subject is singular, the verb must also be singular, and vice versa; this is called 'subject–verb agreement'. In the disjunction between subject and verb, the action and the subject or the subject and the verb do not agree.

In interpretation, the analyst speaks from a non-egoic place, an example of the disjunction between subject and verb, which is a form of bad grammar. In interpretation, the analyst says 'things as it is', instead of saying 'things as they are'. 'As it is' refers to words, gestures, and actions that touch the Real. Verbs and the subject/signifier speak from the place of non-self, and this is one of the meanings of unconscious being structured as a language.

It is to the extent that "symptoms can be read" that "they are inscribed in a writing process" and have no signification in themselves but are, rather, "structured in relation to a signifying structure that determines them" (Lacan, 2006, p. 371)

Out of this structure the subject acts out the holes in the Symbolic, or the lack in the Other, in the form of symptoms or ego-syntomic character traits.

Fenichel (1945) said that neurotic symptoms are ego-dystonic and cause suffering while ego-syntonic character traits are pleasant for the subject but not for others. It is the lack in the Other, or the Other's ego failing, that generates anxiety and depression in the subject. This Lack in the Other appears in the form of grammatical orthopedics that bring a signifying structure to bear on the symptom. The signifying structure generates new signifying chains for the lack in the Other. The Name of the Father (NoF) is always involved in unconscious signifying chains.

Poetry, as metaphor, at first helps us know what to do with the symptom (*savoir faire*); however, this effectiveness is limited by the general knowledge about psychoanalysis in the culture. The symptom, after Freud, becomes a form of jouissance outside language. The symptom as jouissance needs to be transformed into a benevolent Other jouissance (not the jouissance of the m/Other) in analytic treatment and in the final Lacanian theory.

Explanations and comprehension (psychoeducation) are appropriate only at the beginning of analysis or as needed. Interpretation has also been related to the practice of finding and generating meaning polysemically, or secondary meaning, or additional meaning in the patient's speech and material. Although plays on words, such as homophony, equivocality, metonymy/metaphor, and neologisms, are generative semantically, Lacan considers wordplay aimed at generating meaning a failure of technique, leading to more and more symptomatic meaning bound to a bad infinity within the Imaginary.

For Lacan, homophony, polysemy, and slips of the letter, among other forms of wordplay, have no inherent meaning or value as symptoms: the symptom is an excessive form of jouissance that must be brought to a stop in analysis, not by interpreting the symptom and deciphering the meaning behind the letter, but by taking the letter in its material instance (as littorality, or the border between water and land, emotion and the letter/thought) and generating a return to speech from there. But the point is that the substance of expression is only a semblance of jouissance contained within the letters.

Interpretation in Lacan is always addressed to the experience of jouissance and the symptom. In fact, Lacan does not have a theory of interpretation that would understand parapraxes and wordplay as anything more than a satisfaction of the drives. In *Seminar V*, interpretation is the response of the analyst to the analysand's signifying chain and to key signifiers of jouissance, in which case the analyst's intervention would aim to interrupt the analysand's assumed coherence, not to replace it with a new, reconciled meaning, but to maintain attention on the signifiers that structure jouissance.

This was Lacan's version of Freud's manifest and latent contents: whatever manifests symptomatically is to be interpreted not for meaning but for the material differences it introduces through the repetition of the symptom. When the symptom reoccurs as an accident, it is an opportunity (tyche) to do something different with it. The later Lacan interprets jouissance in an analysand, for example, with a gentle gesture on the face of the analysand, saying a word that sounded like the word of a trauma suffered by the analysand.

Indeed, this is why the classical Lacan of the middle period treated the symptom as a metaphor while the late Lacan turned increasingly away from interpretation as wordplay and meaning and toward the interpretation of the signifiers that structure the symptom and the surplus jouissance it generates. Treating the symptom as a metaphor of speech is interesting and makes for interesting conversations but proved to be therapeutically ineffective. This facilitated the rise of cognitive therapy out of the obstacles encountered by psychoanalysts who failed to break out of the bad infinity of the Imaginary relation to which they fall victim as a result of their own ignorance (*Avidyā*) of the nature of psychoanalysis.

The Formula for knowledge about Truth

| Semblance | | Enjoyment |
|---|---|---|
| | $\frac{a}{S_2} \rightarrow \frac{\$}{S_1}$ | |
| Truth | | Surplus Enjoying |

The *a* makes the signifier function as a semblance, as both an appearance and a reality, not a duality of appearance and reality, and a source of enjoyment. According the diagram, truth is outside the Other or knowledge. Surplus enjoyment, rather than enjoyment with a master ego, is an enjoyment of the master signifiers.

Lacan mentions that Georges Bataille, during Lacan's time, gave a lecture in total silence as a form of transmitting non-knowledge. Lacan uses this example to distinguish between knowledge and truth. Truth is silent or revealed in silence. In the text *The Knowledge of the Psychoanalyst*, Lacan plays with all his symbolic formulae and 'mathemes'.

Lacan always lays his foundation in the history of philosophy, as he does with the history of science. He uses both as a tool of interpretation in the practice of psychoanalysis. Of course, that this is theory rather than interpretation. People often complain, 'So what? What does this have to do with clinical practice?'

So how do we translate Lacan's theories in his seminars to practical interpretations and interventions in analytical sessions? In fact, in the practice of analysis, we use the theory to invoke the analysand's material, not to engage in intellectual debates or disputes.

Lacan mentions that Aristotle (2015) places four categories against one another. There is the possible, which Aristotle pits against the impossible, and the necessary, which he pits against the contingent.

What does this have to do with the practice of psychoanalysis? The possible is not what brings people to analysis, unless they are narcissistic and they want to impress the psychoanalyst with what they have already achieved or know. The necessary is what brings them to treatment to satisfy their needs with social goods and relationships. However, the satisfaction of desire is impossible with the satisfaction of need. The mercantile object of exchange appears to offer the impossible good (*objet a* as a *lathouse*) that temporarily satisfies desire but requires new objects to replace these objects unless desire is left unsatisfied. By clarifying what is at stake in the search for the impossible, the analyst helps analysands have the self-confidence to find new relationships in contingent encounters. But then the contingent first refers back to the possible, or the beginning of a relationship, but also leads to the structural and logical end out of the pressure of the necessary. For example, in medieval and modern culture, marriage is socially necessary.

Leibniz's ([1914] 1988) monad or One is part of a structure of four, according to Lacan: monad, dyad, triad, and tetrad. What is the one? Is it a philosophical concept or an experiential concept of oneness or unity? Obviously, it is both, but for psychoanalysis, oneness is not a conceptual but an experiential concept. Each individual is a monad in relationship to other monads. Each individual is a unit reflecting other unities in the universe. The '*indivitrad*' (individual) comes in a structure of four, according to Lacanian theory. Each individual is 1, and is 2 (a divided subject), and is organized by a triadic oedipal structure, and is resolved by a structure of four that includes a new Name of the Father and the Sinthome (holy person).

The Real is affirmed in the impasses of logic; although there are no fissures in the Real, the Real is a plenum. The plenum of the Real can be revealed only by contradictory or paradoxical logic.

In logic, for example, the inverted letter ∋ means that there is a realm of relative particulars. The absolute contains the particulars or the relative, but the absolute or the universal lies at the level of the impossible and at the level of a practice of non-thinking, and the relative lies in the area of divided activity and ordinary thinking. Can these two be in contradiction with one another? For example, the subject works in analysis but does not change in their relationships and everyday life. Or the person meditates but cannot apply the meditation to everyday life.

Lacan looks for a logic that bypasses the principle of contradiction. There are two logics: the principle of contradiction and the principle of non-contradiction. The principle of contradiction is considered not logical or illogical, and the principle of science of non-contradiction simply means the principle of formal logic. However, the principle of contradiction is not illogical or irrational. Leibniz ([1914] 1988), in the *Theodicy*, made this very clear. 'Theodicy' literally means "justifying God" and is a specific branch of theology and philosophy that attempts to reconcile the existence of evil with the belief in a good and all-powerful God.

For example, how did St. Augustine (1950) explain early on the existence of evil if G-d and creation are good and beautiful? Evil as a lack is not a Thing. Augustine argued that evil isn't a separate entity or substance created by God, but rather the absence or corruption of what should be good. Cain is the corruption of Abel, his good brother. In Lacanian psychoanalysis, not accepting the lack may lead to the bad, and accepting the lack leads to the Law. St. Augustine believed that God, being inherently good, could not have created evil, and that the world and everything in it is fundamentally good.

Augustine used the concept of privation to describe evil, meaning that it's the lack of something good that should be present, like darkness being the absence of light, or blindness being the lack of sight and insight. However, this form of duality of good and evil, like that of light and darkness, is a Western concept.

In the East there is also light in darkness, but it should not be treated as light, and there is darkness in light not to be seen as darkness. The privation of light means the existence of darkness and chaos, but light also comes out of the void of darkness. In light, absence or emptiness is not denied but rather revealed. The presence of emptiness reveals the light.

So why does the good need not evil but the localized bad? Well, in the book of Job of the Jewish Tanakh, G-d creates many obstacles for Job in order to develop his spirit through suffering. So the purpose of suffering or of demons or the devil is to serve G-d and realized fulfillment. Christ represents the ultimate obstacle to realize. This is the principle of contradiction and the dialectic of the good and the bad. Was it good or bad that Jesus was crucified or that he became Christ? The good is non-dualistic because good and bad are a duality underneath the overarching good. Sometimes you make mistakes on purpose in the service of the Good.

Lacan follows Parmenides' saying that 'There Is Oneness.' *Yad'lun* and *Il n'ya pas*, or there is the One not of Being, but of the Real as non-being. The One's own non-being: Being is empty in its own being. We access this Real through doing something that appears impossible.

| **Discourse of the Analyst** |
|---|
| $\frac{a}{S_2} \rightarrow \frac{\$}{S_1}$ |

In the discourse of the analyst, we separate the left side of the formula from the right side. This at first may seem arbitrary to others. We locate the analyst on the left side of the formula, and the analysand on the right side of the formula. The first equation, $a/S_2$, represents the analyst relating to the other equation, of the divided subject ($) over $S_1$, which represent the nuggets of speech of the analysand. As you know, there are various types of logical relationships between the terms. The *a* is both the object of the transference of the analysand and how the analyst experiences their jouissance, and what they become in analysis. What they become in an analysis is a product of the fact that in their own personal analysis, they perceived their analyst in the place of an *objet a* in the Real, as indicated in the formula.

The $S_2$ here means not the symbolic Other, or knowledge, but unconscious or unknow-knowing, or the experience of truth behind the experience of the analysis. $S_1$ is the key signifiers that the divided subject unconsciously produces. In analysis the formations of the unconscious are manifestations of the One. At the same time, the analyst represents the One of the unconscious that will make the Being of the analysand possible. In this seminar, Lacan clearly distinguishes between reality and the capitalized Real.

Lacan says that his theory that guides his analytical practice is a philosophical discourse made with the material provided by science, although psychoanalysis is not a science, according to Lacan. That could only be waited for, hoped for. Psychoanalysis is an enlightened delusion, like all theory, and we are waiting for this delusion to bring forth a true science. We could be waiting for a long lime! For Lacan there is no progress, and what we are waiting for isn't necessarily what we will be getting (*on recueille*).

In our opinion, the late Lacanian theory is a holistic theory closer to existentialism and Eastern thought. The subject is divided, as in Freud, but the ego of the Real of the later Lacan provides a new synthesis and a new form of the experience of Oneness.

## Transference as the Stabilization of the Negative

In psychoanalysis, transference emerges as the site where negativity (lack, non-identity) is structured rather than erased. In Lacanian psychoanalysis, 'the dialectic of desire' refers to the idea that our desire is fundamentally shaped by the desire of the 'Other', meaning that what we desire is often driven by what we perceive as being desired by someone else, creating a dynamic in which our desire is constantly mediated and influenced by the symbolic order and the expectations of others around us; essentially, our desire is not entirely our own but is formed through a complex interplay with the desires of others.

It is through transference that desire articulates itself—not as a fulfillment of positivity, but as a sustained movement within lack. In transference love, the subject feels fulfilled, but this cannot last for any changes in the subject to be sustained over time. The analysand does not encounter the lack of and in the analyst until the termination phase of analysis. The problem appears at first to be with subject's own lack, but in the end, the fundamental problem is the lack of and in the Other.

Fulfillment as a positivity is only found in the negative dialectic. In attaching to the analyst, the analysand seeks to be happy, but with negativity and analytic frustration, the analysand recovers the loss of the object as their own subjectivity. Grieving leads to acceptance and gratitude and to transformations of jouissance.

'No' here means a 'yes' that cannot be stated. For example, as in the case of Mahayana Buddhism discussed in a chapter of this book, it is written in the Heart Sutra that in meditation there are

> No feelings, no perceptions, no formations, no consciousness; no eyes, no ears, no nose, no tongue, no body, no mind; no color, no sound, no smell, no taste, no touch, no object of mind; no realm of eyes until no realm of mind-consciousness; no ignorance and also no extinction of it until no old-age-and-death and also no extinction of it; no suffering, no origination, no stopping, no path; no cognition; also, no attainment.
>
> (San Francisco Zen Center, n.d.)

"No feelings" actually means compassion, which is not a feeling. "Formations" signifies the formations of the unconscious; "no taste" means wonderful taste, like the taste of manna from heaven. We don't extinguish ignorance because ignorance also means non-knowing, etc.

The analyst's position is not to negate negation (as in a Hegelian synthesis, or efficiently to repress rather than undo the repressed) but to sustain the negativity in such a way that the analysand can articulate their desire in relation to the Law. In this sense, transference stabilizes the negative: it does not resolve it but allows it to speak about desire. Is this any improvement on the first principle of undoing repression? Freud said he changed his theory to the so-called topographical model to focus on the repressive unconscious in order to increase the effectiveness of analytic practice.

What is negativity, then? Is it denial, conscious suppression as an element of structural repression? What is denied? Is it wishing, the drive, or desire, or all of the above? Freud describes this as when the subject says, "No, I never thought about that." Incidentally, Freud also uses 'negation' to refer to disavowal, whereby in perversion the Name of the Father is rejected or minimized.

French psychoanalyst André Green when he wrote *The Work of the Negative* (1999) to explore how people cope with loss and absence. Green examines how Freud's theories relate to the "work of the negative." He argues that the ego develops against a background of loss, and highlights how accepting lack can lead to new experiences and relationships.

The Life drive is affirmative. Negation is the negation of desire, and the synthesis is the sublimation or the sublation of desire. Now, in negative dialectics the positive is not something that can be affirmed. The positive has only to be affirmed through the negative. So to say that something is, you have to say first that something is not. For example, is a dog civilized like a human, or is a dog uncivilized and a form of the animal instinct? To civilize the dog, you have to negate some of the behaviors of the dog and reward others. Then that becomes the positive—the dog becomes nonaggressive and kind, but he cannot say it in words, he can only show it with signs.

The change of direction toward non-identity is the hinge of negative dialectics. All the formations of the unconscious are forms of non-self and non-identity, not ego, although the ego is unconsciously formed.

The problem with Adorno's dialectical materialism is that there is no Real in it. The Real is outside the Borromean knot and yet it structures inner consistency. The Real is a logically consistent form of the One although it is beyond logic and thought. Negative dialectics is an anti-system and anti-philosophy form of philosophy. It attempts by means of logical consistency to substitute for the unity principle as a philosophical question.

Negative dialectics, as distinct from dialectical negation, does not negate anything because emptiness/void is beyond positive and negative. In negative dialectics, 'no' is 'yes' because the yes cannot be said in words.

However, duality and binary logic are also necessary despite their limitations, because this is how the structure of matter is organized. Yet the human spirit is dialectically organized. A subject may feel both dead and alive while alive, at the same time as dead is dead, and alive is alive. If you have a pulse and breath, you are literally (not metaphorically) alive, not dead.

## Elaboration of the One

If negativity is stabilized in transference, then speech itself becomes the movement of elaboration of the One—not as a totalizing unity but as the singular trajectory of the subject's engagement with lack.

The One here is not the Hegelian Absolute but rather the singular structuring of the subject's speech and desire through the negativity that transference sustains. What does it mean that transference is sustained through negativity? Do we mean the negative transference, or the resistance to analysis? Lacan says that the resistance of the analyst is resistance to letting go of being the Subject Supposed to Know. Transference—its presence or absence—sustains the analyst in the position of non-knowing and favoring the analysand's production of knowing in their speech.

The Absolute for Hegel (1977) is a self-aware "Absolute Spirit" which unfolds through history, with human consciousness gradually coming to know and participate in this absolute knowledge through art, religion, and ultimately, philosophy. Essentially, the Absolute is a spirit that represents the complete and unified totality of reality, where thought and Being are ultimately One. In Hegel there is no awareness of the Absolute as a word not for consciousness but for the unconscious.

Remember that for Lacan, the One is the One's own non-being. One stems from zero as the first number. In Lacanian theory, the Absolute is more like a Real emptiness. What Hegel considers as the Absolute is actually the historically relative knowledge of philosophy.

## Psychoanalysis and Negative Dialectics

The psychoanalytic situation is not dialectical in the Hegelian sense (where negation leads to a higher synthesis). In Freud, negation can lead to sublimation, but sublimation for Freud is not a form of the negative or repression. The drive is not transformed through repression, because repression is a direct expression of the Death drive.

Adorno's insists that negation should not be resolved into a reconciled unity—transference stabilizes negation without sublating it. Negation is itself a form of sublation. In this sense, analysis aims not at knowledge-as-synthesis but at sustaining the speaking subject within negativity, within the speaking about loss and lack of the object.

This presents the transference as a space of sustained negativity, which contrasts with many interpretations of analysis that assume it is about insight or meaning-production. Instead, analysis is about maintaining the structural conditions for desire's articulation, allowing the analysand to continue speaking without reducing their speech to a fixed resolution, although their suffering or jouissance may be transformed.

Psychoanalytic practice itself is an ethical practice of negative dialectics, in which the task is not to reconcile contradictions but to sustain the conditions for their elaboration.

The Real, as a hole/whole, is a unity outside the Symbolic and yet constitutes what coheres and holds the Symbolic together. This refers to what Freud said regarding the difference between analysis and synthesis in response to Assagioli (1971), the inventor of psychosynthesis, a supposedly New Age and humanistic perspective. Freud said our ego did not introduce meaning (in contrast to Frankel, 1949) into the experience of the patient. Coherence comes from unconscious synthesis or takes place unconsciously. Discourse is the discourse of the unconscious, or of the unconscious ego, not of the ego, something that Freud ambiguously stated in the *Metapsychology Papers* and then reversed in *The Ego and the Id*, indicating a theoretical regression, according to Lacan.

What kind of unconscious works according to synthesis? Is there a harmonious unconscious? Lacan answered first no with the division of the subject, but later yes with the Real that makes accord in a new structure. Freud said that the unconscious rather than the synthetic ego performs syntheses, perhaps similarly to a computer. I propose that unity and synthesis can be Imaginary or Real, healthy, or pathological.

Lyotard (1988) and 'post moderns' rejected the idea of a conscious humanistic synthesis or harmony, or a synthetic ego, although they were not aware of unconscious synthesis that take place for the good, as Freud believed. Unconscious synthesis does not follow a conscious humanistic scheme, as is the case with humanistic ideology and many of its critics. Unconscious syntheses operate silently and effectively. Assagioli critiqued Freud for neglecting synthesis, which Freud believed happened naturally, unconsciously, and did not have to be guided by the analyst's values. Assagioli (1971) disliked theory and thought it was a question of how it is applied, by whom, and to whom. He rejected theory that included an ontology and axiology he did not like.

The concept's unfolding (of analytical elements relating in a new way) is also a reaching back, and synthesis is the definition of the difference that perished as a mistake, 'vanished', in the concept. Only in the accomplished synthesis, in the union of contradictory moments that don't lose their moment of contradiction, will their difference be manifested. Without the step that Being is the same as nothingness, each of them would be indifferent to the other; only when they are to be the same do they become contradictory (Adorno, 2000, p. 157).

The One is grounded in difference or the Many (the power of the people), not in sameness. Striving for identity leads to the suppression of difference, while the acceptance of difference leads to an experience of a singular identity for each individual or '*indivitrad*'.

"The One begins with the lack" (Lacan, 2018, p. 126). The monad is that by which each entity may be said to be 1; and number is very precisely this multiplicity composed of monads.

Number is *nad* in Spanish, which leads to the word 'number' as *nad* or *nada* (nothing). This is the same as the term 'cipher', which also means "number" and "zero" in Sanskrit. While the English word 'cipher' originates from the Sanskrit word '*śūnya*', meaning "empty" or "zero", and the Arabic word "*sifr*" (also meaning "zero"), the Sanskrit word '*śūnya*' itself is the direct equivalent of "zero" and does not have a meaning of "number" or "coded message". However, in number theory, zero is the beginning of number, and not 1.

Number is multiplicity composed of monads. 'Monad' is the term by which an entity (a quartz, atom, molecule organs, bodies) may be said to be One. One is also, Lacan says, a bag with a hole in it. *Yad'lun*, or 'there is of the One', is the master signifier.

Freud felt repugnance for universal love. As a Jew, he understood that loving one's neighbor meant loving a fellow Jew, not a Christian non-Jew with whom he experienced mutual strangeness. While Jesus in Christianity universalized love for all humanity, for Judaism, if each relative group loves each other as themselves, then eventually in the end of time that will become a universal love.

Then, while wisdom in Lacanian theory is knowledge of jouissance, isn't love a type of jouissance, and does it not provide the emotional stability for a school of Wisdom?

In this seminar, Lacan changes how he interprets the Cartesian "I think, therefore I am." Instead of the imaginary conscious ego thinking and self-creating itself, Lacan says, "'*Ca se pense*' or 'It thinks itself', therefore I am." It is the unconscious that thinks (thoughts without a thinker), not the conscious ego. The conscious is a semblance that simply repeats the parrot empty speech. But for the late Lacan, we need to listen to this repetitive parrot speech, because there is an enigmatic meaning in its truth.

According to Lacan, there is no existence of the One other than in mathematical existence. However, Lacan contradicts himself: in *Seminar XX* he talks of feminine jouissance, and of the jouissance of the mystic as forms of the Real. Here Lacan disagrees with himself, and I disagree with him.

In a moving final moment, Lacan shows his vulnerability rather than his mastery when he says,

> I never dropped any of the people I knew were going to leave me before they left of their own accord. And this is true also of the period to which I alluded a moment ago when the match was lost for France, the little brouhaha Amid plotting by the medically qualified psychoanalyst, which gave rise to the start of my teaching in 1953.
>
> (Lacan, [1971–72], p. 173)

This points to the fact that his teaching started and ended with conflict; he did not believe there was any progress in this regard in groups or society in general. Justice as a principle is 'just what is', or how things are, usually murky and unclear. However, when the ethnic masses of the poor are welcomed by the goddess of liberty to America, this principle provides a source of respect for the host country and for each other. Isn't this progress? Wasn't the French Revolution progress? Not if we consider that the revolution gave birth to Napoleon—but then Napoleon, despite his hubris and final death, gave the new citizens their individual rights in their country. Human rights became a symbol of progress and modernity.

Lacan gave his students his human rights, but it was they who abused him and were in conflict with him (not because he was a despot?). Lacan, more than Freud, wanted to believe in humanity, but like Freud he died in disappointment, although lucid about the drive for repetition and destruction that cannot be subdued despite religion and culture.

The barred subject is the subject in as much as it is nothing other than the effect of the signifier. However, this nothing, I have argued, which the subject is, is a form of jouissance according to my argument. "I am 'This'." 'This' is not an object but a form of bliss without an object.

In *Seminar XVI, From the Other to the Other*, which was not previously translated by Cormac Gallagher, Lacan thinks of the Other in terms of set theory. If inside the A, as a symbol/image of a circle, as symbol of a set, in set theory, there is no element a as an element but rather we find $S_1$, $S_2$, $S_3$, etc., we say that the A is not an element of itself for the signifier. The A/a is outside the signifier. Does the big Other not exist as a signifier? What about the word 'Other'? Here, like a mirror, the Other is empty, in contrast to the other of our brother and neighbor. $S_1$ and $S_2$ are elements of the big Other. Is the Other, as the structure of language, not in the signifiers? Signifiers are elements of the Other, but the Other or its structure are not signifiers. Some key signifiers and their structure are unconscious, both in a real repressed sense and in non-thinking sense.

For Lacan, the I of the ego, not the subject, demands the ego from you, or from the Other/other. I desire what you desire, and ... I demand myself ... what you desire.

When Lacan addresses Pascal's wager, there are four terms in relation to one another: two small *objet a*'s, 0 in two places, and Infinity. What do these terms mean? Lacan does not explain them or define them in this seminar.

Lacan says that rather than giving an exact formula or being a mathematician, he prefers a discourse without words which designates that discourse as sustained by writing, which Lacan mostly did not do. Writing is done in silence. Lacan wrote the *Écrits* early on, followed by decades of oral seminars, and he ended the last seminars silently looking at the blackboard instead of at his audience, as he had done for years. This was interpreted as a sign of his old-age dementia, although he was still respected as a genius and people attended his seminar to watch him stand there in total silence not-thinking.

We know that somewhere in that part that we call the unconscious, the truth is uncirculated, like signifiers circulate through metaphor and meronomy. Here there is evidence for two forms of the unconscious. One is repressed, and the second is unsymbolized and Real and its property is that we cannot know anything about it. We may ignore this Real, or we may non-know it.

We wrote that knowing about the function of truth minus knowledge should give us the truth about knowing. We have to find truth without too much knowledge. Truth minus knowledge leads to a critique of the literature and prior knowledge. Does this mean that truth is only silence without knowledge? Silence here leads to innovation and new knowledge.

Science consistently excluded what is mystical about the idea of knowledge; it renounced this knowledge to constitute a knowledge that is an artifact handled by the subject. Moreover, the subject can be purified to be only the support that articulates ordered knowing. Either unknown-knowing or knowledge is a discourse that is separated from public opinion (Doxa), and that distinguishes itself as being the discourse of science.

The subject supposed to knowing is G-d, and that's the extent and end of the story, according to Lacan's Christian theism!

Lacan didn't say that the Other doesn't know. He said that the place of knowing is the unconscious, only it is not a subject. The negation in the formula that there is no Subject Supposed to Know falls on the subject, not on knowing. The subject does not know; only knowing knows. Who is it that knows? Who knows who they are? Who or what is this subject? This subject cannot be known or said, only spoken as the word 'self' or 'myself'. However, this supposition facilities the emergence of true knowledge and being yourself, despite there being no-self.

## References

Adorno, T. W. (2000). *Negative Dialectics*. Translated by E. B. Ashton. Continuum: New York.

Aristotle. (2015). *The Organon*. London: Bloomsbury Academic.

Assagioli, R. (1971). *Psychosynthesis: A Manual of Principles and Techniques*. New York: University of New York Press.

Etchegoyen, R. H. (1991). *The Fundamentals of Psychoanalytic Technique*. London: Karnac Books.

Fenichel, O. (1945). *The Psychoanalytic Theory of Neurosis*. New York: Norton & Norton.

Frankel, V. (1948). *The Unconscious God*. New York: Simon and Schuster, 1975.

Green, A. (1999). *The Work of The Negative*. London: Free Association.

Heart Sutra. (2025). https://www.sfzc.org/files/daily_sutras_heart_of_great_perfect_wisdom

Hegel, F. *Phenomenology of Spirit*. (1977). Translated by A. V. Miller, Oxford: Oxford University Press.

Lacan, J. (1953–1954). *The Seminar of Jacques Lacan*. Book I Papers on Technique, 1953–1954. New York: Norton and Norton.

Lacan, J. ([1968–69] 2023). *From the Other to the Other. The Seminar of Jacques Lacan, Book XVI*. Translated by B. Fink. London: Polity Press.

Lacan, J. ([1971–72] n.d.). *The Seminar of Jacques Lacan: The Knowledge of the Psychoanalyst 1971–1972*. Translated by C. Gallagher. n.p. http://www.lacaninireland.com/web/translations/seminars.

Lacan, J. ([1971–72] 2018). ... *Or Worse*. The Seminar of Jacques Lacan, *Book XIX*. Translated by A. R. Price. London: Polity Press

Lacan, J. (2006). *Écrits*. Translated by B. Fink. New York: Norton.

Lacan, J. (2018). ... *Or Worse*. Book XIX. London:n Polity Press.

Lacan, J. *(1953–1954). The Seminar of Jacques Lacan. Book I Papers on Technique, 1953–1954*. New York:Norton and Norton.

Lacan, J. *(1953–1954). The Seminar of Jacques Lacan. Book I Papers on Technique, 1953–1954*. New York:Norton and Norton.

Leibniz, G. W. ([1914] 1988). *The Theodecy*. Cambridge University Press.

Lyotard, J. F. ([1979] 1988). *The Postmodern Condition: A Report on Knowledge*. Translated by G. Bennington and B. Massumi. Minneapolis: University of Minnesota Press.

Moncayo, R. (2017). *Lalangue, Sinthome, Jouissance, and Nomination*. London: Karnac.

Peirce, Charles S. (1955). *Philosophical Writings of Pearce*. Edited by J. Buchler. New York: Dover.

San Fransisco Zen Center. (n.d.). *Heart of Great Perfect Wisdom Sutra*. https://www.sfzc.org/files/daily_sutras_heart_of_great_perfect_wisdom

Vasubandhu (1984). *Seven Works of Vasubandhu the Buddhist Psychological Doctor*. Edited by S. Anacker. Delhi: Motilal Banarsidass.

Wittengstein, L. (1958). *Philosophicaln Investigations*. London: Wiley-Blackwell, 2009.

Wittgenstein, L. (2002). *Tractatus Logico-Philosophicus*. Translated by C. K. Ogden. London: Routledge & Kegan Paul. Originally published as "*Logisch-Philosophische Abhandlung*", in *Annalen der Naturphilosophische*, XIV (3/4), 1921.

# 2 The Five Discourses Plus One

What is the difference between the knowledge of a psychoanalyst, that of a teacher in the university discourse, and that of a spiritual but not ideological teacher of knowledge? Lacan's theory of discourse is another attempt to formalize the knowledge of the psychoanalyst with 'mathemes' or symbolic formulas that organize the work of psychoanalysis and its relationship to culture and politics. Žižek has written a lot about this topic, not being a practicing psychoanalyst himself.

The practice of psychoanalysis is a talking cure for the analysand and a listening practice for the analyst. The patient is supposed to free-associate and speak freely without holding anything back. There's no discussion of politics or elections or taking sides in the patient's conflicts with their family. This is why psychoanalysis speaks in the language of science and politics speaks in the language of imaginary ideology.

Now, what do ordinary people believe about discourse? I think people believe that language is important for social communication, and they learn language in their relationship with their families and teachers in school, where they learn about intellectual topics. So, what Lacan calls 'discourse' refers to intellectual and scholarly discussions among teachers and students, scholars, and politicians.

University discourse is not the same as the master's or government discourse. An intellectual discourse may not emerge in the university like psychoanalysis, for example, but then is either rejected as not scientific or is researched and proved efficacious by university discourse, which then authorizes the mental health system's insurance to pay for it.

In this sense discourse is always related to power, to those to whom we speak, and to what position we are in as parent and child, teacher and student, colonizer and colonized, capitalist and worker, or leader and subject. Here I present to you the four discourses.

DOI: 10.4324/9781003658702-2

| **Discourse of the Master** | **Discourse of the University** |
|---|---|
| $\underline{S_1} \quad \underline{S_2}$<br>$\$ \quad a$ | $\underline{S_2} \rightarrow a$<br>$S_1 \rightarrow \$$ |
| **Discourse of the Hysteric** | **Discourse of the Analyst** |
| $\underline{\$} \rightarrow S_1$<br>$a \quad \underline{S_2}$ | $\underline{a} \rightarrow \underline{\$}$<br>$S_2 \rightarrow S_1$ |
| **Discourse of the Capitalist** | |
| $\underline{\$} \rightarrow \underline{S_2}$<br>$S'_{1.} \quad a$ | |

## Terms and Definitions

$\$$ = the divided subject or psychical *Spaltung*.

$S_1$ = the master signifier, of which there are two: first, the signifier of the master; second, the signifier when the signified is in the body of jouissance. The true master teaches with their body.

$S_2$ = the signified in language and in a dictionary.

*Objet a* = the object cause of desire and there are seven imaginary objects total: breast, feces, phallus, hole, voice, gaze, and the 'nothing' or the agalma that is in the Real.

So far, I have been speaking of discourse as an intellectual capacity, but Lacan also speaks of discourse as a form of jouissance. Now, jouissance is not a feeling but represents the pleasurable and painful aspect of feelings. Truth for Lacan always represents something enjoyable, but truth could also be painful to bear. The master is a transcendent ego that conforms to the myth of the ego ideal that dominates our actions. In this sense, the university discourse and the master's discourse always form a type of 'egocracy'. Here Lacan speaks of G-d as jouissance, more like the Buddha in Buddhism, rather than like the Jewish God of the superego and the Mosaic Law.

The formulas include four terms that are in various logical relations to each other, of alternation, opposition, and subjugation. $S_1$ is the signifier, and $S_2$ is the signified or signification in language. S or $\$$ is a divided subject. For Lacan's psycholinguistics, the subject is the same as and is defined by the signifier. The *objet a* is the object cause of desire. *Objet a*'s are imaginary and real (agalma), while the signifier is symbolic.

As the discourse of the master or of the government can be seen as ordinary life, the discourse of the hysteric could also be called the discourse of psychopathology or the discourse of suffering.

Finally, the discourse of the capitalist is the discourse wherein the subject completes themselves through consumption and science, and knowledge about the objects of consumption also leads to increased consumption. Lacan calls the *objet a* a '*lathouse*' to refer to the use of computers, internet-based information, and AI to impact consumption and economic exchange. The information about the *objet a* is imaginary, but it facilitates economic exchange. The value of the good life is more satisfying than is the pleasure afforded by material goods, although the two work together. The use value or labor value of the object is not its jouissance value, which cannot be measured in rational numbers. The imaginary number (symbolic, for our purposes) represents the happiness value of productive human activity. Jouissance value is measured in irrational and complex numbers.

Does the theory of discourse in Lacan's theory have the notion of religion as represented in the theory of discourse? Is religion a master's discourse with God being the master? Lacan reduces religion to a form of social link that can also be expressed in the secular form of language. There is also Lacan's distinction between the God of the Law and the G-d of jouissance or of mystical jouissance or bliss. The G-d of jouissance is the G-d of spirituality, of a spiritual teacher, not a political master.

I said above that Lacan also speaks of discourse as a form of jouissance. Now, jouissance is not a feeling but represents the pleasurable and painful aspect of feelings. Truth for Lacan always represents something enjoyable, but truth can also be painful to bear. The master is a transcendent ego that conforms to the myth of the ego ideal that dominates our actions. In this sense, the university discourse and the master's discourse always form a type of 'egocracy'.

This egocracy is not the same as the discourse of the master or $S_1$. In other words, there are two forms of the $S_1$, as I have indicated before (Moncayo, 2017). However, Lacan puns on *maître* as the master of unbeing or *désêtre*. Roudinesco (1994) says that this is Lacan's own undoing of his mastery rather than a culmination of his ego of the Real. She sees it this way because he was a member of the communist party and had no spiritual perspective.

But this is spiritual mastery, like Freud saying that self-mastery is a fruit of a personal analysis. But Freud's master is a strong rational ego, not a sadistic superego, while Lacan's form of self-mastery is non-egoic or of the subject. There is the $S_1$ of the master, as in feudalism and the master–slave dialectic. The master is courageous, but the slave is hardworking but fearful of freedom.

The slave is a collectivity—for example, the masses—while the master is an individual all-alone amidst the collectivity yet not lonely. The subject of the Real is all-alone and is master of only themselves, not of others, and does not depend on the social recognition provided by others or the social Other. The true master is not a master of others, but the true teacher is not an ordinary school or university teacher either. Again, the discourse of a spiritual teacher is not a university discourse and is also not a religious ideology used to influence voters, like religion is.

What is the difference between a teacher in the university discourse and a spiritual but not ideological teacher, or a teacher of knowledge? Knowledge in psychoanalysis is knowing rather than based on theory. Unknown-knowing comes from the personal experience with the unconscious. The psychoanalyst is a teacher of non-knowing as a form of Eastern and Western wisdom.

## References

Moncayo, R. (2017). Lalangue, Sinthome, Jouissance, and Nomination. London: Karnac.

Roudinesco, E. (1994). Lacan. Mexico: Siglo Ventiuno Editores.

# 3 The Ethics of the Lack in Psychoanalysis

One thing is the theoretical knowledge of the psychoanalyst, while practical ethics focuses on what can be hoped for in analytic treatment. Practical ethics in psychoanalysis is not the morality of licensing boards or the moral boundaries of the psychoanalyst.

The concept of ethics is a philosophical one, in contrast to morality, which is a religious concept, although not exclusively so. One of the aims of psychoanalysis is to perform a rational or scientific analysis of morality, and this is part of the study of ethics. The knowledge of the psychoanalyst aims to understand the concept of unconscious guilt. This to be distinguished from conscious remorse, which is more rational and can be undone.

A key concept of ethics and morality is that of pleasure. The concept of pleasure includes both the pleasure of the good and the good of pleasure that might not be ethically good. Lacan ([1959–1960] 1986) posits the ethics of desire, as opposed to an anti-desire form of morality. Do you live consistently with your desire as a subject? The only thing you should feel guilty about is having given up on your desire.

Rather than repress unconscious wishes, sublimate them, and adjust them to reality, following Hegel, Lacan invents the concept of desire based on lack. We should live in reality according to our sublimated desire, not repress it or deny it. Desire and the Law make you a subject of society and the unconscious. Freud considered guilt pathological and unnecessary, but Lacan allows it in relation to desire. Erich Fromm (1947) called it humanistic guilt that leads to personal growth, as distinct from instinctual desire.

Spinoza's *Ethics* ([1961] ), for Deleuze, constitutes a rejection of the transcendent Good/Evil distinction in favor of a merely functional opposition between good and bad. The transcendental Good and Evil lead to the sad passions.

The ethics of psychoanalysis according to Freud, ego psychology and object relations.

Freud believed that analysis leads to self-control and self-mastery. The analytic frame is also a container for fantasies that don't get acted out in reality. The frame is consistent with the incest prohibition. Analysis also leads to a transformation of the pathological aspects of morality and repression in favor of rationality.

DOI: 10.4324/9781003658702-3

Ego psychology sees this as linked to the ego, which transforms the drives and the primitive process. Object relations develop an ethic of care and concern and of good enough mothering. These are maternal aspect of psychoanalysis as opposed to the father-oriented Freudian psychoanalysis, which does not have these concerns. A father can be remote and absent and still function as a father. The mother also has to be a symbolic mother, make herself absent, and accept the orifices within herself. The analysis of the function, rather than recognizing the role of the father in the family, is very important for psychotherapy and psychoanalysis.

Rationality is not considered by Lacan as an ego function. Rationality is the order of the structure of language and society ordered by Law. Its representative in the personality is the subject divided between signifier and signified, between material substance of expression and signification and meaning.

Lacan distinguishes among *Sashe*, or the object; *Wort*, which is the word; and the thing or 'no-thing', which is *das Ding*. In Chinese, one word means both 'word' and 'thing'. 'Thing' is related to nature, and 'work' is related to culture, but China is a culture rooted in Nature.

*Das Ding* is outside signification and is different from drive. The no-thing represents the existence of the void in the center of the Real. *Das Ding* is another name for the *objet a* in the Real.

Jacques Lacan's ethics of desire is based on the idea that desire is ethical and that the only guilt one can have is for giving up, not for giving in to one's desire, as in traditional morality. Lacan believed that desire is the root of ethics and that the moral law is desire in its purest form. How can pure desire be a desire for the pure Law if ordinary human desire is a desire to transgress the Law?

Desire is ethical: Lacan believed that desire is ethical because it is the subject's good. However, Lacan distinguished between the good of desire and the desire for the good. Both goods are not the same. Guilt for Lacan is a betrayal of desire: Lacan believed that guilt is a result of betraying one's desire, not a result of breaking a moral rule. Desire is also a desire to know. Lacan believed that desire is valid only if it is a desire to know. Desire is desire for being or unbeing; desire is an object of loss. Lacan believed that desire is an object of loss, which is why we want it.

For Žižek (1989), the ethics of psychoanalysis are based on the Lacanian ethical framework, but Žižek's ethics are critical of postmodern liberal multiculturalism. Thus, *the ethics* is, for Deleuze, an 'ethology', that is, a guide to obtaining the best relations possible for bodies, which is also descriptive of racial and cultural difference.

## The Ethics of the Lack

Is ethics ideology, or can it be used as ideology and hypocrisy? We know that ideology is fantasy, but what about ethics? The issue of ideology as false beliefs and values refers to two phenomena: the use of morality to disguise immorality and the use of morality and beliefs to defend and protect the economic and political positions and privileges of those in power. Often illusory power is taken from others, and the immorality of the act is disguised as an attack on the other's morality and ethics.

In addition, the Marxist concept of ideology could be enlarged to include any use of ideas, values, and beliefs to protect and defend the economic interests of any given individual or class. One could say that this only applies to a society based on scarcity and classes. But even in socialist societies, power structures and elites have to compete to enter university or this or that profession, compete for this or that position within an institution, such as a political party. It is these vital interests or desires that introduce distortions and biases into the conceptions of reality that men and women have.

Perhaps psychoanalytic theory can be helpful in trying to understand how basic needs and desires play a part in an unconscious process of ideological distortion and delusion. Freud taught us that moral values are rooted in the id and the unconscious. In other words, in my view, not only is there a duality between moral duty and wishful impulses or drives such as sex and aggression, but that there is an actual dialectic between them.

Dialectically, rather than dualistically, there is impulse and wish within morality, and there is morality within wish and desire. Let us turn our attention first to the impulse basis of morality, which Freud tried to explain scientifically rather than by divine commandment. Freud thought of morality as developing or arising in a process of reaction formation or of turning a drive into its opposite. Morality is developed by identification with the moral will of the parents, and this identification replaces id object-cathexes that have been abandoned. Hatred or hostility toward the parent is suppressed by strengthening the opposite feeling of love through an identification. This identification not only has the function of desexualizing the love felt toward those in authority but also has the social function of promoting the acceptance of social norms and behavior.

In addition, the subject will not only love paternal and maternal figures and their ideals but will then turn the aggression felt toward to the parents toward themselves and toward others who, like themselves, may wish to violate the law of the father/mother. Thus, this is how wish is turned into duty, hate into love, and sexual love toward the parents into social and sublime 'neighborly' love. Furthermore, throughout this process of transvaluation and transformation of psychical values, love is turned into a more refined product than craving, immediate self-centered gratification, lust, and the kind of love that leads to destructive attachments associated with envy, greed, and jealousy.

Now, the critical point for our discussion is that because good and bad are interrelated, mutually arise, and refer to each other in unconscious ways, morality/religion as 'ideology' (false belief) can be used to express opposite values. Altruism can be used to express egoism, and vice versa. People can cover up to others and themselves their true interests, desires, motivations by reaction formations, by acting as if, for example, they were motivated by the disinterested desire to help others.

This is an interesting point because the very mechanism that morality, society, and religion use to transform the base and destructive inclinations of human beings into the opposite can also be used to disguise these impulses and to serve their ends. It is indeed often difficult to separate enlightenment from delusion, altruism from egoism, morality from the id, ideology from science, appearance from reality, false views and beliefs from true views and conceptions, liberation from domination, and so on. Such separation depends on context and usage. A slight twist or difference can make all the difference in the world.

I mentioned earlier that in a dialectical view, not only are there primitive drives within morality, but there is also morality within desire. Primitive drives can be expressed through morality, or morality can be used to cover up destructive or forbidden ulterior intentions, but morality also serves the ends of or is an expression of a desire that is not necessarily primitive or destructive. Thus, we say that ethical ideals are wishes, hopes, dreams, and aspirations of humanity. And thus, there is something utopian about morality itself—a paradox indeed.

On the one hand, morality serves the establishment of a social reality principle; on the other hand, morality articulates an idealistic (not actual or factual) aspiration or potential yet to be fulfilled.

Within psychoanalytic theory, the normative and restrictive aspect of morality is attributed to the agency of the superego, while the 'libidinal' aspect of morality constitutes the positive side of the superego known as the 'ego ideal'. The energetic basis of the superego has to do with aggression, while the energetic basis of the ego ideal has to do with libido or desire.

In Freud's theory, the concepts of identification and sublimation are interrelated because in identifying with the moral will of the parents, the child's desires toward these parents are also transformed. Instead of wishing an impossible physical union (whether pre-genital or genital) or a destruction of the parent, these impulses are sublimated in the direction of ethical ideals. In the process, energy is transformed qualitatively from a free-restless state to a quiescent state. In addition, object libido is transformed into ego or narcissistic libido, hence the term 'ego ideal'.

Certain desires will now have to be satisfied intra-psychically via the ethical ideals of the ego. Nevertheless, there is a basic desire that remains constant throughout these changes. And my point here is that there is something intrinsically moral about this desire.

Freud saw the origin of morality as being intrinsically related to the formation of defenses within the structural development of the mind. In fact, defenses were considered to be early precursors of morality. Freud associated the repressive force with a principle governing the functioning of the nervous system: the Nirvana principle. In his view, the nervous system (and the mind) strives toward a lowering or a possible elimination of painful nervous excitation, or what now would be called 'stress'. This is part of the brain–mind relationship and how it relates to ethics.

The first example of this principle can be observed in intrauterine life. The fetus exists within the body of the mother in a well-balanced environment with respect to nutrition, temperature, and the exclusion of external stimuli. It is a metaphor for the Garden of Eden, where needs are met without regard for time or space or the existence of a subject and an object. The body of the child is a part of a larger body. Thus, we could say with Plato that desire already knows about a previous world or a possibility of utopian or ideal satisfaction and balance. This original balance will be disrupted by the process of birth and the arrival into a world of time and space, of separate subjects and objects.

Lacan considered the division or heteronomy of the subject with respect to the signifier. Lacan's permutation of the Cartesian cogito ('I think where I am not') describes the subject's passivity with respect to the activity of the signifier. Thinking and the signifying chain proceed of their own accord. The subject of experience, which has identified and internalized the cultural laws of language and the language of cultural laws, is a spectator, an observer, a voyeur with respect to their own thought. This is the division and duality between language and a subject in the world.

The subject has been socialized to speak according to the rules of formal, logical, grammatical language; yet from this perspective, the subject becomes alienated from their own desire and thought, which acquire an 'autonomy' from the subject. Where should heteronomy and autonomy be located? In the coercive structure of formal language granting autonomy within the law (of language which is isomorphic with cultural laws), or in the incessant stream of thoughts which the subject cannot control? How can the subject of the Real reach non-thinking as the state of truth?

For Freud and others, this latter solution had long ago stopped functioning as such and instead had become part of the problem. However, lest the subject produce a psychotic decompensation, the bounds of formal conventional language can never be completely dispensed with. The social Other of conventional language will always remain a necessary reference. It is part and parcel of being in an unavoidable world of duality and division.

Nonetheless, the autonomy of desire, wishful thinking, and the signifying chain also provide an imaginary solution. Habermas located the source of emancipatory autonomy not in the conflict-free spheres of ego functions but in the utopian fantasies and dreams of the id. Yet Lacan has taught that desire itself is intrinsically and dialectically linked to the law of symbolic castration. Hence, although internally autonomous with respect to external social culture, desire inherently remains determined by the psychical law of castration. Symbolic castration compels one to desire in the mold of a hedonistic, defensive, obsessional formation.

Here we can avoid the romanticism of the id that runs through Feuerbach, the young Marx, Reich, Loewen, Guattari, Laing, some aspects of the Frankfurt School, and so on. Instead, we follow the line that goes through Freud to Marcuse and Adorno. We can say that Lacan picked up the line after Freud, and that this line continued through Deleuze and the next generation of Lacanians.

Moreover, it is important to remember that, technically and clinically speaking, desire is usually linked (bound) to imaginary heteroerotic and autoerotic, hetero-aggressive and auto-aggressive fantasies. The objects of desire are generated within these fantasies. The phantasm to which desire is attached has the function of denying castration. However, the illusory escape from castration's grip demands that the subject pay the price of remaining bound and fixated to the phantasm. From this perspective, it becomes possible to envision the limitations of any utopian id-romanticism. Marcuse stands out from this group with his concept of repressive and non-repressive desublimation.

If not in the heteronomous tyranny of the signifier and language, and not in the autonomy of desiderative thinking, where can the autonomy of the subject be found? What about the autonomy of ego-identifications? Is autonomy the wish to do what the social other wants from you? Desire as the desire of the Other or the Law or Name of the Father translated into learned socialized behavior? In this model, autonomy would be based on independently desiring what your parents desired from you as a child. The acquisition of sphincteric control in early childhood provides an accurate 'posterior' metaphor.

Acquiring basic rules of cleanliness and socialization grants the individual independent freedom of movement within the social world. And so we land squarely back on the classical, conventional notion of freedom within the bounds of the law, freedom within social form. Is this social autonomy or being a social automaton? At least in constriction and coercion there is no illusion of freedom, but in choosing the Law, the subject is granted an illusory egoic space of depicting social behavior as voluntary.

Is autonomy limited to the subject choosing the law of their own free will? Perhaps the way out of this dilemma is a consideration that the concept of choice is too soft a notion. More than chosen, the Law needs to be won, acquired, and rediscovered by each and every subject, by each and every generation. This leads to understanding what Aristotle meant by arguing that the potential of human nature is acquired through the actualization of social culture.

For example, when utilizing social language, the *moi*, the ego, says, 'I think, I speak'. This is the illusion of ego autonomy. Moreover, the I is a reaction formation against the tyrannical or coercive nature of the signifier. Numerous 'I thinks' are within the track of goal-oriented thinking, of goals and objectives, of anxieties about what will I become at the level of an ego-representation. But here, where I think I am, in the *moi*, am I not being instead an imaginary object of desire of the social other, of my parents, their dreams and frustrations? In line with this, Lacan (1972) permutates the Cartesian cogito 'I think, therefore, I am' to 'I think where I am not'. It is desire as the desire of the other that is doing the thinking activity. I am being lived by the dreams and desires of many generations before me.

Therefore, one level of psychoanalytic emancipation (autonomy) is reached through finding the 'not-me' within the symbolic pathways of desire. 'I think where I am not' is transformed into 'I am where I do not think', in the sense of 'I am' where it is not the I that is doing the thinking. I am merely a toy of desire within the signifying chain. This sense of me is what Lacan calls the subject of the unconscious that can be won, realized, and reappropriated in the practice of analysis. However, a further, larger 'I' still needs to be reached beyond the pathways of symbolic desire on the level of emancipation and autonomy corresponding to the authentic spiritual function.

'I am where I do not think' signifies the realm of being beyond signification and representation alluded to in prior chapters: our real self, the Big I that is beyond thought and that is capable of saying, "I am This I am" (Exodus 3:14). I am a form of jouissance and samadhi (Sabbath bliss). Thus, through psychoanalytic practice the subject can find, realize, and reappropriate their own symbolic identity within the laws of desire and language, but the subject is also capable of doing the same with respect to the emptiness of absolute identity.

At this juncture, autonomy and heteronomy become the same non-dual thing. Jung (1939) referred to the 'autonomy' of unconscious contents in the same way that Lacan refers to the heteronomy of the signifier. Nevertheless, once the heteronomy of the real and symbolic registers is repossessed, then the so-called autonomy of these worlds becomes the autonomy of a centered subjectivity without a subject.

Thus, we are not transforming the heteronomy of the Symbolic and the Real into an imaginary ego-based autonomy; rather, the 'heteronomous autonomy' of these registers is transformed into an 'autonomical heteronomy' of the subject: heteronomy because no-self signifies that multiple processes, elements, and conditions provide the context for a subject, but autonomy because when no-self is actualized then all things advance the self, or all things become the activity of our Big self.

When the subject becomes benevolently depersonalized, then the question of who is speaking becomes an important way of conveying or denoting the meaning of selfhood within both the Symbolic and the Real. Is such autonomy or heteronomy? This paradox cannot be resolved completely by language or formal logic. The symbolic self of social reality has been given a particular individual embodiment within a subject, yet such conventional autonomy also must pass the test of Nature as revealed through the subject. 'Nature' here means not only the id of passion and desire but also the It as the expression of a natural will through the formation of a second nature derived from a synthesis between nature and the general social will.

In this case, for example, the mature autonomically heteronomous subject may differ from conventional social law. John Dewey (1932) noted that higher morality also requires collisions between conventional authority and liberty. Liberty within the Law is not the same as freedom from the Law. But here it is important to note that there is a difference between what can be called the democracy and autonomy of the Id and the democracy and autonomy of the It. The first is the rule of passion, of Nature and of drive. The second is the rule of a second-order nature that in Buddhism is called Buddha nature. Ethics or the precepts, that emerge from Buddha nature. In a similar way, in Judaism, the Torah, or the Law, emerges from G-d in a revelation.

In Kabbalistic fashion, the word 'liberty' can be permutated by backward spelling and homophony into the word 'It-rebel'. Ideological forms and social knowledge need to interact with and pass the test of what Barthes ([1953] 1968) called the biological reality of discourse. The Socius (the social symbolic body) not only must be embodied and reappropriated by its subjects but also has to pass the test of Nature as expressed through a single subject who may be at odds with social convention but at one with reality in the wider sense of the term. Social forms need to be verified and confirmed within experience, and the latter includes the register of the Real as a nonconventional, extra-social, and transhistorical nature beyond symbolization.

According to Piaget ([1932] 1997), higher morality requires that parental and societal rules be subjected to the critical test of reason and reciprocity: are social laws reasonable, and are all individuals equal before them? In this light, it is possible to regard all three agencies of Freud's so-called structural theory as representing potential forms of autonomy before the law. There is the autonomy of desire, of the rational ego, and even of the super-conventional or religious superego. However, none of these forms would encompass the phenomena of liberty in terms of a differing impulse emanating from 'It'. For emancipation, in its ultimate spiritual sense, subjectivity must not only be liberated from false ideology in the Marxist sense (this is how Habermas defines a rational emancipatory critical interest) but must also spring up from the register of the Real beyond social language and thought.

Traditional practices such as meditation and the Jewish day of rest lie beyond rational, political, social-critical practices to the extent that they have a justification outside the arguments of reason; they go beyond ideology since they are essentially not based on ideas, discursive thinking or a field of strategic goals and objectives. In addition, although Habermas defines critical reason as different from instrumental reason, the latter is part of the former because critical reason is always concerned with the strategic goal of attaining social and political power. This is a contradiction because apparently Habermas is not aware that there are two different forms of reason. The ethics of reason are united with Sophia as a love for knowledge for its own sake. The goal of attaining power is karmic and represents a distortion or regression of Phronesis to Techne.

*The Ethics* for Deleuze is not only the creation of a plane of immanence but also the creation of a whole regime of new concepts that revolve around the rejection of the transcendental in all spheres of life. The unity of the ontological and the ethical is crucial for Deleuze—in understanding Spinoza, that is.

Spinoza didn't entitle his book *Ontology*—he's too shrewd for that: he entitles it *Ethics*. This is a way of saying that whatever the importance of my speculative propositions may be, you can judge them only at the level of the ethics that they envelop or imply.

In short, as the title of one of Deleuze's books, *Spinoza: Practical Philosophy*, indicates, *The Ethics* is understood only when it is seen, at the same time, to be both theoretical and practical. Deleuze considers there to be three primary theoretico-practical points in *The Ethics*: "The great theories of the Ethics… cannot be treated apart from the three practical theses concerning consciousness, values, and the sad passions".

First of all, the illusion of consciousness. Spinoza argues that we are not the cause of our thoughts and actions but only assume that we are based on their effects upon us. This leads to dualisms of substance (such as Descartes' mind/body split). Deleuze insists on this point because he sees Spinoza bypassing an important illusion of subjectivity: we suppose that we are causes and not effects of the Other of language and the unconscious.

The illusion of consciousness, for Spinoza, is a result of inadequate knowledge and sad effects, allows us to posit a transcendental consciousness supposedly free from the interventions of the world (as in Descartes). This is, in fact, a blind spot that precludes us from knowing ourselves as cause, the practical meaning of which is that we deny our own 'sociality', as one mode among others, and the significance of the relations that we enter into, which actually determine our power to act and our ability to experience active joy.

Then comes the critique of morality. Spinoza's *Ethics*, for Deleuze, constitutes a rejection of the transcendent Good/Evil distinction in favor of a merely functional opposition between good and bad. Good and Evil for Spinoza, as for Lucretius and Nietzsche, are the illusions of a moralistic worldview that does nothing but reduce our power to act and encourages the experience of the sad passions. *The Ethics* is for Deleuze rather an incitement to consider encounters between bodies on the basis of their relative 'goodness' for those modes that are relating. The shark enters into a good relationship with salt water, which increases its power to act, but for a rose bush, salt water only degrades the characteristic relations between the parts of the bush and threatens to destroy its existence.

So, actions have no transcendental scale to be measured upon (the theological illusion), only relative and perspectival good and bad assessments based on specific bodies. Thus, *The Ethics* is, for Deleuze, an 'ethology', that is, a guide to obtaining the best relations possible for bodies.

Finally, Deleuze sees in Spinoza the rejection of the sad passions. This point is linked to the last, and again closely related to Nietzsche's critique of resentment and slave morality. Sad passions are for Spinoza all those forces which disparage life. For Deleuze, Spinoza denounces all the falsifications of life, all the values in the name of which we disparage life. We do not live; we only lead a semblance of life; we can only think of how to keep from dying, and our entire life is a death worship.

The hinge that this practical reading of Spinoza turns on is Deleuze's angle of approach to *The Ethics*. Rather than emphasizing the great theoretical structures found in the first few sections, Deleuze emphasizes the later part of the book (particularly part V), which consists of arguments from the point of view of individual modes. This approach puts the importance on the reality of individuals rather than form and on the practical rather than the theoretical. In the preface to the English translation of *Expressionism in Philosophy*, Deleuze writes, "What interested me most in Spinoza wasn't his Substance, but the composition of finite modes… That is: the hope of making substance turn on finite modes, or at least of seeing in substance a plane of immanence in which finite modes operate…" (p. X).

Deleuze's reading of Spinoza has clear and profound relations with all that he wrote after 1968, especially the two volumes of *Capitalism and Schizophrenia*.

## References

Barthes, R. ([1953] 1968). Writing Degree Zero. Translated by A. Lavers & C. Smith. New York: Hill and Wang.

Deleuze, G. ([1969] 1990). Logic of Sense. Translated by M. Lester with C. Stivale. New York: Columbia University Press.

Dewey, J. (1932). Ethics. Carbondale: Southern Illinois University Press.

Fromm, E. (1947). Man for Himself. New York: A Fawcett Premier Book.

Jung, C. (1939). Archetypes and the Collective Unconscious. Princeton University Press: Bollingen Series XX.

Spinoza, B. ([1961] 1980). The Ethics. Translated by G. H. R. Parkinson. Oxford University Press.

Lacan, J. ([1959–1960] 1986). La Etica del Psicoanalisis. Buenos Aires: Paidos.

Lacan, J. (1972–1973). ...Or worse. The Seminar of Jacques Lacan. Book XIX. London: Polity Press.

Lacan, J. (1972–1973). ...Or worse. The Seminar of Jacques Lacan. Book XIX. London: Polity Press.

Zizek, S. (1989). The Sublime Object of Ideology. London: Verso Books.

# 4 Triads and Quaternities

Continuing with knowledge, in mathematics and arithmetic, the first number is either zero or one depending on the number system and the cultural historical reference. Every number is a unit/trace, and in contemporary mathematics, zero is included in each number of set theory.

In a unary number system, starting with zero, three is the fourth number.

In the natural number system, without a zero concept, three is the third number.

Three is the third cultural number needed to mediate the natural biological relationship between mother and child are a binary two. So then there's a question of cultures that begin with zero (Indian) and cultures that begin with one (Europe). Zero-based cultures are based on the values of negation and renunciation and compassion and of love for the other. One-based cultures are based on love of the individual I and the ego, as is the Renaissance.

## The Other Third in Hegel's Dialectic

In formal logic, a proposition is either true or false. The false helps arrive at the true, but without constituting a truth in itself. In probability theory, the truth only represents a probability that a proposition has a percentage of being true. In order to be true, a proposition has to be at least 50% true, or at least a half-truth and a half-fiction.

For formal logic, a fiction is something false, while for dialectical logic, a fiction is a form of truth or can lead to truth. In dialectical logic, the truth is a third element as a form of synthesis. In negative dialectics, the synthetic element falls off, and what takes its place is the negative that includes the positive without saying it.

Negative dialectics drops the ambition of dialectical knowledge of gaining or achieving an absolute form of knowledge, which is not falsifiable because its truth remains not in the relative Symbolic but in the different order or dimension of the Real (truth of jouissance). Jouissance as truth can be relative (fusion with the mother), phallic (intercourse), or absolute: the third Other jouissance.

DOI: 10.4324/9781003658702-4

In Hegel there are three elements in knowledge: thesis, antithesis, and synthesis. The third element synthesizes the previous two into a new proposition. In the negative dialectics of Adorno, the synthetical element disappears because consciousness does not produce synthesis; only the unconscious does as I have argued. In this sense the unconscious represents a more legitimate, therapeutic form of knowledge.

In quantum theory, energy waves in the void generate both particles and identical antiparticles with reverse charge that are not synthesized except that in rare occasions the positive particle is not destroyed, and matter is created out of its replication and differentiation. This is not a dialectic.

## The Third in Peirce and Linguistics

For Peirce, the interpretant or interpretation of a sign/representation is a second representamen or representation. The first or primary representation for Peirce represents an object, the meaning of which is given by a second representation/signifier. For Peirce, semiosis is a triadic process. The first is a signifier or representation, the second is the object in the world, and the third is the element of interpretation, or interpretant. In Peirce's Triad, there is 'no-thing' in itself, in contrast to Lacan. For Lacan, the object world is produced by the signifier, and the thing itself remains outside the signifier.

For Peirce, the object and the interpretant are two correlates of the sign, the one being antecedent of the sign, the other consequent of it. The problem with Peirce's theory of the sign is that it conceives of an original relation between the sign/representation and the object, as if the sign had derived from a quality of the object instead of the signifier determining the meaning of the object world.

## Freud's Metapsychology

Freud's metapsychology is composed of the unconscious, preconscious, and conscious. At first the unconscious was the repressed, and the repressive force was conscious. The preconscious was unconscious in a descriptive sense although not repressed, and consciousness always has an object of sense and Sense (meaning) that constitutes a determined form of consciousness. There is also the less known awareness, which refers to the magical writing pad that has no code and no memory and is a clear pathway for knowledge to become internalized and subjective. Awareness does not have memory or code.

## The Structural Theory: Ego, Id, and Superego

Freud was not satisfied with the therapeutic results of the first metapsychological theory of undoing repression in analysis and making the unconscious. He then focused on undoing the defenses that he came to understand as also unconscious but not repressed. The source of repression he attributed to an unconscious part of the ego, but he could not resolve how this differed from an unconscious superego as the source of repression. The unconscious superego can also suppress the unconscious ego in Freud's theory. This is the negative or destructive aspect of the Death drive. But the Death drive is also what cancels/castrates the subject in favor of the subject as a form of non-self.

## Jung's Theory

Jung divides the mind/psyche into collective unconscious, the personal unconscious, the ego, and the Self. According to Jung, woman is the fourth of the Christian trinity: Name of the Father, the Son, the Holy Spirit, and woman. For Freud, there was no personal unconscious because the individual unconscious is simply a partial identification with the collective Other. Speech and images speak through us. The concept of Jungian androgyny is like Freud's concept of unconscious bisexuality; however, androgyny differs from sexual difference and the concept of symbolic castration.

## Lacanian Theory

Lacan's uses the repressed unconscious, the descriptive unconscious, and the Lacanian Real unconscious. The Real unconscious appears in two forms: the first Real is dreadful and destructive, and the second Real creates harmony or accord. The second Real is what Lacan calls the name of the father emerging from the Real and the *sinthome*. Bion (1995) also has the 0 similar to both of Lacan's Real but not so much the Other of the symbolic unconscious.

When the analyst renounces to be in the place of the ideal and does not respond to the demand of the analysand, then in that void the analysand's fundamental fantasies will become apparent. The analysand not only wants the analyst to tell their what to do or not do—a demand for a demand—but also demands that the analyst give their the signifier of the phallus as well as the object of love and of the drive. Finally, the analysand also wants to become and give the analyst the object that the analyst desires, lacks, and needs. The analysand wants the analyst to demand this object from their, but the analyst refuses to do so.

Following Lacan, I will use the permutations of the Cartesian '*cogito ergo sum*' to illustrate the three dimensions of the subject. 'I think [I speak], therefore I am' represents the self-image and the imaginary ego. When utilizing social language, the *moi*, the ego, says, 'I think, I speak'. As Fink (1997) has pointed out, when the ego says I speak, "What he means thus refers to a level of intentionality that he views as his own; it refers to an intentionality that fits in with his self-image" (p. 24). This is why Lacan made a conceptual distinction between the enunciating ego and the subject of the enunciation and between meaning and signification. Meaning is imaginary because "it is tied up with our self-image, with the image we have of who and what we are". Instead, the subject of the unconscious, of the Symbolic, of signification, and of the enunciation is conceived by Lacan as an effect of the operation of the signifier. The classical Freudian slips, the parapraxis, the double meanings, the polyvocal significations, in short, all of the formations of the unconscious are effects of the language-like symbolic structure of the unconscious.

Within a Lacanian framework, it is the symbolic order (a set of laws, values, myths, etc.) and the order of language that establish the structures and functions of the subject that in the ego-psychology school are attributed to non-defensive and 'realistic' ego-functioning. For Lacan, reality is a social construct given by the culture-bound and law-bound order of language. The rules of language and the rules of kinship (i.e., incest prohibition) are conceived as two fundamental and integral elements of culture. In addition, the Other refers to parental figures and figures of authority from whom the subject receives both social rules and the rules and content of language. Just as the ideal ego and narcissism are derivative objects of the desire of the mother, so it is the relationship with the symbolic father that frees the subject from narcissism and from being an imaginary object of the mother's desire. The identification with the symbolic father establishes the subject as a pivot of the Symbolic and the Symbolic as a pivot of subjectivity.

Lacan's second Real generates a new ego and a new unifying principle where meaning can be enigmatic and beyond words. Finally, a third permutation of the Cartesian cogito brings to the fore the third dimension of experience: the register of the Real. The symbolic 'I think where I am not' needs to be permutated into 'I am where I do not think', which I interpret as signifying the realm of being or parabeing beyond thought, signification and representation.

## Personality as a Subset of Mind

Let's start by defining Mind as distinct from the ego, although personality theory is also understood as a branch of psychology or of the theory of Mind. It is important to stress that Freud had a theory of Mind, because otherwise the ego and the personality could simply be understood in behavioral terms as conditioned behavior or as an aggregate of stimulus and response packets under the heading of habits.

Personality for Jung was the social mask. For Lacan, the person is *personat*, or a personal or sounding through or hearing (*Jouis-Sense*). Jung focused on sacred images, while Lacan focused on the Symbolic/Real sound. Now, it is interesting that sound is linked to phenomenology and yet to the most efficient structural causes that can be counted with one hand. What you see is not how you see it. A phenomenon is replaced by structure precisely in the moment of the suspension of nonessentials. Structure is a function of the essence, which is emptiness.

Freud identifies the conscious part of the ego with the seat of reason. However, there is more than one type of reason, and this is something that Freud did not consider at least in a systematic way. The aspect of the ego that functions according to ego-representations, narcissistic investments, and aggressivity conflicts with the impartiality associated with reason in science. But the awareness and pure intellect associated with preconscious perception of the external world would in fact be consistent with the principles of science. However, the unconscious intellect also knows things intuitively. *Nous* or the unconscious intellect provides the axioms, which then must be tested by consciousness. Fantasies or fictions are generated by the fantasized ego.

Lacan's new ego or subject of and in the Real is a fourth-degree differentiation within narcissism. This is the rock of symbolic castration and the most difficult of narcissistic wounds: the symbolic father and phallus are also found to be lacking, a zero or a nothing. Once the illusions regarding the ideal father and the disillusions regarding the lack and limitations of the father have been cleared in the transference to the analyst, the father remains as an empty symbolic function but a function nonetheless. There is some similarity here with Jung's Self, which is a Hindu concept, while Lacan's subject is similar to the Buddhist notion of no-self.

The final Lacan argued that the subject is an 'answer of the Real' and not 'an answer of the Other' or of the Symbolic. However, the autonomy of the subject is empty or devoid of any inherent meaning. It is only within the Imaginary that the ego imputes to itself the function or agency of generating new meaning. New meaning is generated within the Symbolic itself as a function of the interaction between the emptiness of the Real and of the subject and the dynamic interaction between the elements of an open structure under ongoing construction. You have to fly the plane while it is continuously being constructed and improved. You have to use the self although there is no-self. Conventional egos and professionals have a difficult time doing precisely this.

## References

Bion, W. R. (1995). Attention and Interpretation. New York: Jason Aronson.

Fink, B. (1997). A Clinical Introduction to Lacanian Psychoanalysis. Cambridge, MA: Harvard University Press.

Freud, S. ([1893–1895] 1966). Studies on Hysteria. New York: Avon Books.

Freud, S. (1914). On Narcissism: An Introduction. In: *The Standard Edition of the Complete Psychological Works of Sigmund Freud*, Volume 14. Edited by J. Strachey. London: Hogarth Press, 67–102.

Freud, S. (1923). The Ego and the Id. In: *The Standard Edition of the Complete Psychological Works of Sigmund Freud*, Volume 19. Edited by J. Strachey. London: Hogarth Press, 3–66.

Jakobson, R. (1990). On Language. Cambridge, MA: Harvard University Press.

Kohut, H. (1966). Forms and Transformations of Narcissism. *Journal of the American Psychoanalytic Organization*, 14, 243–272.

Lacan, J. ([1957] 2006). The Instance of the Letter in the Unconscious. In: Ecrits, translated by B. Fink. New York: Norton.

Lacan, J. ([1958–1959] 1970). El Deseo y su Interpretacion. Seminar VI. Edited by O. Masotta. Buenos Aires: Nueva Vision.

Lacan, J. ([1959–1960] 1992). The Ethics of Psychoanalysis 1959–1960: The Seminar of Jacques Lacan, Book VII, edited by J. A. Miller, translated by D. Porter. New York: Norton.

Lacan, J. ([1960] 2006). The Subversion of the Subject and the Dialectic of Desire. In: Ecrits, translated by B. Fink. New York: Norton.

Lacan, J. ([1972–1973] 1998). On Feminine Sexuality, the Limits of Love and Knowledge 1972–1973: Encore: The Seminar of Jacques Lacan, Book XX. Translated by B. Fink. New York: Norton.

Lacan, J. (1975–1976). Book XXIII. The Sinthome: The Seminar of Jacques Lacan, Book XXIII. Cambridge: Polity Press.

Moncayo, R. (1998). Evolving Lacanian Perspectives for Clinical Psychoanalysis: On Narcissism, Sexuation, and Jouissance in Psychoanalysis and Culture. London: Karnac.

Moncayo, R., & Romanowicz, M. (2015). Going Beyond Castration in the Graph of Desire. *The Letter: Irish Journal of Lacanian Psychoanalysis*, 58, 31–58.

Nasio, J. D. (1992). The Concept of the Subject of the Unconscious. In: Cinq Leçons sur la Théorie de Jacques Lacan. Paris: Rivages.

Porge, E. (1997). Los Nombres del Padre en Jacques Lacan. Buenos Aires: Nueva Vision, 1998.

Roudinesco, E., & Badiou, A. (2012). Jacques Lacan, Past and Present. Translated by J. E. Smith. New York: Columbia University Press.

Winnicott, D. (1970). The Maturational Processes and the Facilitating Environment: Studies in the Theory of Emotional Development. London: Routledge.

# 5 The Philosophical and Psychoanalytic Concept of History

Now, one may ask what does history have to do with knowledge in psychoanalysis? History is known as a series of past events that has an intrinsic pattern or structure. Most people use 'history' for the next bad thing to come, or what you don't want to happen to you. History always returns to the same bad thing. Usually, history documents politics, governments, wars, and change. History also points to the future, insofar as people want to make the future a better place for the new generations.

In psychoanalysis, 'history' refers to an individual's past experiences, particularly those from early childhood, which are believed to significantly shape current thoughts, feelings, and actions and which can be accessed and analyzed through the analytic process to understand unconscious desires and structures. Essentially, a person's 'psychical history' is considered crucial to understanding that person's present struggles and problems.

'Psyche' or 'Mind' here means how a person's narrative history builds the structure of their mind. However, this happens across two dimensions of time: synchronic and diachronic. 'Diachronic' is not necessarily as a form of growth and development; the mind could also end with a chaotical structure, as in psychoses. 'Synchronic' here means all the elements of the structure appearing at once in a moment that elevates the subject to the wider level of the non-thinking mind. The Psyche also manifests in two levels, unconscious and conscious. The conscious is the story and narrative telling, and the unconscious manifests in the unconscious signifying chain.

The unconscious in psychoanalysis emphasizes the role of repressed memories and conflicts from early life that continue to impact present behavior, even if the individual is not consciously aware of them. Freud's psychosexual stages of development (oral, anal, phallic, genital, latency) are pivotal in shaping personality and are often examined in psychoanalytic psychotherapy. The stages of development are part of the diachronic or the historical dimension of time.

Through the analytic process, individuals may reexperience past traumatic events and fantasies, allowing them to process, traverse, and transform these experiences into their current understanding of themselves.

DOI: 10.4324/9781003658702-5

## Psychohistory or Psychobiography

Psychohistory is a field that applies psychoanalytic theory to analyze historical figures and events, attempting to understand their desires and psychological dynamics based on available information. This is also the field of psychobiography. Lacan did not believe that you could interpret without knowing the patient's associations in a session. He did not accept Erikson's biography of Luther and Gandhi. Lacanian theory breaks away from any thematic analysis of a narrative and forgoes a primary reference or analysis of a story based on the psychobiography, childhood experience, or personality of the author. In addition, the narrative of the analysand in analysis is not necessarily interpreted in terms of the social or family history of the conscious subject. The stories that are told and said are analyzed in the logical and emotional terms of the unconscious signifying chain. More than the conscious family narrative, it is the unconscious signifying chain that manifests the truth of the subject.

## Different Views of History

Different philosophers have viewed history in various ways, with some seeing it as a divinely guided process unfolding according to God's plan, while others considered it a progression toward greater human freedom (Hegel, 1774) or a series of repeating cycles of rise and fall (Nietzsche; Eliade, 1949; Cassirer, 1946) across different civilizations.

St. Augustine believed that history is a linear progression guided by God, culminating in the final judgment, with events like the Fall of Adam, the Exodus of the Jews, and the life of Jesus as pivotal points.

Georg Hegel (1770) considered history as a dialectical process moving toward the realization of human freedom, with each stage containing contradictions that lead to a higher synthesis.

The general views are the following:

Teleological view

Many philosophers, particularly religious thinkers, believed that history has a purpose or goal, often tied to divine providence.

Cyclical view

Some philosophers saw history as a series of repeating patterns, with civilizations rising and falling in similar ways. History, in this view, must strive to return or repeat the sacred origin of humanity. The order of instinct (and genetic determination) leads toward the life of reproduction, led by the chaos of nature. Civilizations and the mind are destroyed by this chaos. History is not only the repetition of progress but the repetition of the same problems.

Linear view

Enlightenment thinkers often saw history as a continuous progression toward greater human advancement. This is a modern secularized view of biblical history, for example, of the Exodus, the liberation of the Jew from enslavement. Hegel's (1974) philosophy of history emphasizes the development of freedom and the consciousness of freedom over the course of world history. Hegel does not consider the unconsciousness of the structure.

For development is marked by conflict and struggle, rather than by smooth uninterrupted progress, and is manifested for the most part in political developments construed broadly, including world-historical events such as the French Revolution; in the significant actions of world-historical 'heroes' such as Alexander the Great, Napoleon Bonaparte, George Washington, Abraham Lincoln, Winston Churchill, and Franklin Delano Roosevelt; and in the achievements of peoples and nations.

The period between the fall of the Western Roman Empire (around the fifth century) and the beginning of the Renaissance (around the fourteenth to fifteenth century) essentially marks the 'middle' period of the Middle Ages between classical antiquity and modern times. The middle period is often called the 'medieval' period. Of course, that modern or scientific modernity and democracy originated in a period of history distinct from contemporary society, the postmodern, or poststructural or postcolonial, period.

As we know, 'structuralism' refers to a way of thinking that emphasizes the radical uncertainty of knowledge (particularly knowledge in language) and posits that 'truth' is not a fixed concept but instead constantly changes based on one's cultural, political, social, and economic position in the world. From this 'Foucauldian' point of view, truth in history is always changing, and new forms are destroying and incorporating old forms of history. However, this view ignores the aspect of truth that is universal and outside history and knowledge. In the end, truth in the Real brings the linear concept of history back to the circular, axial, or atemporal concept of time and history. In the end the straight line is a circle.

According to Hegel, the end or goal of history is the actualization of freedom in the life of modern nation-state. Hegel claimed that history was a rational process of development and that it could be understood and made intelligible for anyone willing to look at it rationally, which means looking at it holistically and as an endeavor of the World Spirit with a discernible purpose. However, everybody knows or has experienced the irrationality and passion of history. Irrational numbers are also organized by irrational mathematical numbers.

Here I find a contradiction between human freedom and the World Spirit or will. Is the World Spirit G-d's or the holy human spirit? Only in the convergence or synthesis of the two is the contradiction resolved between the will of the Other and the freedom of the subject. But many in history have perished under this contradiction, either fighting against the Law or fighting against Nature.

Moreover, Hegel attempted to show that history exhibited real progress toward the ultimate goal of freedom and that the modern period, the time in which he lived up until his death in 1831, brought this development to fruition and, in a way, a culmination. His awareness of history pointed to the end of history, like the Bible does. This theory of history has been both highly influential and controversial—it is essential to any overall study of the philosophy of history.

The theory of history reflects Hegel's philosophy and dialectical method. The spirit dominates philosophy and history. A dominant king, or empire, is opposed by another nation with culture and ideals that are claimed to be dominant. Dominance and hegemony are not necessarily bad in that they may promote global development. The dominant country spends a large percentage of its budget in the military to maintain global peace. The United States has been the world's police force, although now this is being challenged. Other nations can then spend money on development and catching up. This is the example of the United States and China: the United States spends money on the arms race, and China focuses on national defense.

China offers a good historical example where the peasants rebelled through armed struggle and oppressed the oppressors. Then, to liberate the workers, the Communist Party established the dictatorship of the proletariat and went through purges of its own officials. Vietnam did the same and entered into a war of liberation with the United States. Now Vietnam is even more liberal than China.

Now, do the people feel oppressed by a dictatorship? Not if it is a form of paternalism and the growth and wealth of the people are emphasized. This is the case for China and Vietnam, but not for North Korea. China's GDP grew at an amazing rate for forty years thanks to free economic exchange and capitalism, not due to state-owned enterprises, as for the Soviet Union, which is no more. The public companies competed with the private sector and thus became more efficient.

So, the two systems combined rather than struggled and opposed one another. This is a good example of the dialectic and of synthesis, which is unopposed by an antithesis and ongoing struggle.

Now, previously, Hegel's student Karl Marx inverted Hegel's theory. For Hegel, the World Spirit is what matters in how it influences a culture. The suprastructure determines the infrastructure, while for Marx, it was the reverse: the infrastructure determines the suprastructure. You can be educated but live in dilapidated buildings and wear old clothes. In this respect, China emphasized how development is maximized through the building of great infrastructure, without too much ideological suprastructure. But without suprastructure and freedom of ideas, China cannot innovate to higher levels of technology, as in the West, despite having the talent. Talent requires innovation and freedom from censorship. The Western internet is censored in China, although now all the Chinese want to be Western with Chinese characteristics, thanks to Deng Xiaoping and Xi Jinping having lifted them out of poverty. Some became richer than others, but that was acceptable.

Hegel saw alienation and contradiction as necessary for development and progress. Culture alienates the animal or instinctual nature and socializes the young against their will. Marx instead interprets this as the dictatorship of the proletariat. The animal spirits must win and repress the divine spirits who exploited them and made them work. Marx did not understand a pure love for work and thought that this did not exist among the working class. But the mind state, or the suprastructure, heavily influences productivity and benevolent excess.

The late Marx saw impersonal bureaucratic structure and organization as necessary, although alienating. In China, such communist bureaucracy worked in harmony with a traditional Chinese meritocracy and bureaucratic state organization. Finally, China did not struggle with America to develop because America helped and benefited from China's development.

Representative democracy unites the common sense of the many with the talent of the one, and this is a universally valid form of government. Talent, meritocracy, and rule by principles and ideas are the best form of government. The best people rule in the service of the people because they possess judgment, courage, justice, and moderation in the highest degree.

Socrates thought that the ambitions that drove most political leaders were a form of madness or a sickness of the soul. This perspective is entirely consistent with Darwin's and Freud's accounts of male leadership in the primal hoard. If justice is equality and rulers should be concerned with the welfare of their subjects rather than themselves, then justice promotes the interests of the weak not the strong, as in the Bible, contrary to the animal spirits.

If we use this analysis to review what happened during the 2024 elections in the United States, we see that Trump's election victory was a victory of the less educated and blue-collar workers over the educated middle class and the educated rich. For years the Democratic Party privileged college education as a path from the working class to the middle and upper classes. However, the less educated felt diminished or left behind by this, plus jobs were outsourced to other countries with lower wages and fewer worker protections.

Trump appears to favor the uneducated working classes, but in fact the working classes are supporting the tax cuts for the super-rich as if they themselves benefit in some way. Trickle-down economics, or voodoo economics, as it is often called, claimed that lowering taxes for the rich would benefit the poor as well.

Trump is a man of no virtue, has been convicted of sexual abuse and assault, and is a narcissistic pathological liar. Even his riches are questionable. His lack of virtue was an advantage with his voters and led him to victory. He is very self-centered and thinks about himself before others. His followers love that vicariously, and think of themselves as members of a superior great nation.

If G-d is the ruler of history, then a gentile with no virtue has to be the anti-leader or the Antichrist. If G-d is not the ruler of history, then such is simply the product of karma, our impulses, and destructive passions. Such a figure does not exist in Judaism. Trump has no virtue, so he cannot be a savior, despite what his followers think. In any case, according to Christianity, true leaders and the messianic world will come after the Antichrist.

What about Trump's support of Christian pro-life, anti-abortion values? Well, Christianity is the only religion that bases its faith on a prohibition on abortion. There's no prohibition on abortion in Judaism or Buddhism. This cannot be a universal value.

The major conflicts between capitalism and socialism have been resolved or reconciled, but what about the contemporary example of Russia and Ukraine?

Russia invaded Ukraine with the imperial ambitions of the old czars and because some Russians living in Ukraine near the border with Russia wanted to be part of Russia. This implies that the fall of communism in the Soviet Union could have led either to liberalism (West Germany) or to the emergence of Russian nationalism. The war is one between autocratic Russian nationalism and a liberal political global order with established and recognized borders ratified by the United Nations.

What about colonialism, a term that has been so vilified in the West? Colonialism is the cultural aspect of an empire. This is something that the Mongol empire, for example, did not have. Their empire was simply based on physical force and numbers. If an empire is not a civilization, then its grip on power will be short lived.

First an empire is built through military innovation. Then the empire imposes or brings their values to their colony. India became English speaking and developed industry and its economy with the help of English values operating in harmony with traditional Indian values. This is why this form of empire is called a 'civilization'. A 'colony' means a settlement leading to agriculture. The earth and animals are our colonized, but they both have developed and been harmed by colonization.

Finally, there is the war between Arabs and Jews in Israel and its role in history. Both people are descendants of the Canaanites, but the Hebrews were made slaves in Egypt and later became Jews. G-d pointed to Israel as the promised land of the future Jews who were living in Canaan. They would go back to Canaan as Israel not as Canaanites, but the other Canaanites and Palestinians remained there and either had to be killed or have their own country.

In this sense, this struggle in history is biblical. G-d promised to Ishmael to make him a great nation but did not promise him a holy land like he did to Isaac's descendants. Both people are still fighting over the same land, but only one people has a right to inherit the land according to the Bible, thought not to history, if these two are not the same.

If G-d is the ruler of history and is not intervening, this seems to confirm the theory that the dominant nation is the ruler of history. In the wars in the

Bible, God is always determining which side will win based on their moral behavior. When Christians fight Muslims and Muslims fight Jews, and all three believe in the same monotheistic God, on which side of the war is God on? If you say the winning side, then there is no way of determining whether the war was won by God or humans. The victors are always the superior cause.

G-d and history seem to be helping Israel with its military technology. For the conflict to be resolved, both peoples need to accept a common border and a Jewish inheritance to the land. Muslims must renounce violence, while Christianity must abandon its claims to religious exclusivity (salvation only through Christ), which the late Pope Francis did. Judaism must also embrace the brotherliness of humans and major religions.

Finally, the cyclical form of history has two views. The first is repetition as trauma, genocide, and the second is general suffering as destiny. This second is Tyche, or destiny, wherein humans struggle in repetitions that are therapeutic and lead to evolution, change, and enlightenment. This view of destiny does not conflict with the view of history and evolution as linear progress. In space, in the end a straight line becomes a circle, so the two views are reconciled.

Now, is history organized by various ideologies and discourses? What is the difference between ideology, science, religious texts, and discourse? For Lacanians, ideology is imaginary and discourse is symbolic. For example, in Genesis, G-d creates the material universe with symbolic words: "Let there be light." The ideology is that G-d is a father in heaven that guides our development. The symbolic discourse is that G-d does this with the Law.

The rule of the king or master in history is the ideological form of the ruler of history or his earthly representative. If you are a Buddhist, for example, then you are guided by ultimate reality or Buddha, but historically, Buddha did not get involved in government or political life. Buddha meditated and watched armies collide in war; he did not try to stop them. How can a sacred, wise consciousness take sides in a violent struggle? From this point of view, how can G-d be the ruler of history?

The master ($S_1$) can be a spiritual master or a governmental or economic master (plutarchy, or the government of billionaires). $S_2$ is the ideology or teaching that is used to rule.

## References

Augustine. (1950). The City of God. New York: Doubleday Books.

Cassirer, E. (1946). Language and Myth. New York: Dover Publications.

Hegel, F. (1974). Lectures on the History of Philosophy, 3 Vols. Translated by E. S. Haldane and F. H. Simson. New Jersey: Humanities Press.

# 6 The Mahayana Teaching of Mind-Consciousness and Freud's and Jung's Metapsychology

In the first chapter, we discussed Mind and Psyche as an experientially unconscious of no-mind and beyond unconscious thinking. Mind is also logical and mathematical in psychoanalysis while being a form of jouissance and emotional truth.

I say 'Mind-consciousness' in the title of this chapter because Mind could be unconscious as in Freud and in Zen Buddhism (Suzuki, 1960; Suzuki, 1970). There are three modes, or fields, of perceptions: direct, as representation, and as mere images. Representations can be in words or images. Images are visual representations.

The first field of perception is the perception of things-in-themselves, or 'as they are' or 'as it is', perceiving directly without distortion or delusion. This may seem scientific and objective, but it is a subjective heart experience. This way of perception is in the realm of noumena, or suchness as distinct from phenomena. 'Suchness' means the goodness of reality as it is. Another name for the Buddha is the Tathagata, which means 'the one who has come from suchness and goes to suchness'.

If while walking in the street you see a dog, your perception of it belongs to the realm of representations.

All images, whether we perceive them in the mode of representations or in the mode of mirror images, are false according to Buddhism. How could reality be false, rather than true and harmonious, as organized by the dialectic of form and emptiness? This is where Joshu, in the Book of Serenity, raises the question of the dog's Buddha-nature and kindness, rather than its animality. The dog has no Buddha-nature, unlike a human, but dialectically, no means yes.

The first five consciousnesses—the sense consciousnesses of eye, ear, nose, tongue, and body—are capable of touching the realm of things in themselves, especially when they contact their objects of perception without the participation and intervention of Mind-consciousness. This is where empiricism in science and psychology derive their effectiveness.

When we see a table, what we perceive as a table belongs to the field of representations not of objects, because our perception has a lot of

DOI: 10.4324/9781003658702-6

Mind-consciousness in it. Intuition is a form of knowing that is not based in thinking and imaging. But intuition is not just spiritual but perceives the unseen or perceived underlying structure of physical and material reality. The structure of the atom is not observable but must be intuitively imagined.

The eighteen elements of perception and being, according to Buddhism, are the six sense organs, their sense objects of perception, and the resulting six consciousnesses.

The objects of mind are thinking, imagination, and ideas. The result is Mind-consciousness.

The three Dharma seals can be categorized into two groups: those that have leaks, and those that are without leaks. Those without leaks are right speech, sitting in stillness, and right actions. Having leaks means that there's still something dripping out, like water from a cracked earthenware jar. It means that the action does not have the nature of true insight and liberation, and there's still the possibility of falling down and turning back from the fruits of our actions. Eating more seeds of delusion in our consciousness without leaks means an action or experience is pure without seepage. Note that I wrote 'seeds of delusion' because there are no seeds of enlightenment. The seeds of enlightenment are when the seeds are realized as empty or nonexistent.

An action will produce wholesome or unwholesome karmic effects when leaking in the world of birth, death, and suffering, the world of Samsara. This is the historical dimension. Phenomena without leaks belong to the world of no birth and no death, Nirvana, the ultimate dimension.

The representational world and language is a mode of false perception. From a cognitive perspective, this would be a delusional view since language and perception as inborn characteristics needed to construct reality.

The sixth consciousness, or Mind-analytical consciousness (*manas–vijnana*), is able to discern the differences among sensations, such as sound or smell and so forth. When our mind-consciousness is able to perceive things directly, it is capable of touching the realm of suchness or so-called external reality The way to train our mind-consciousness in correct perception is through mindfulness. Mind-consciousness, or mindfulness, in this case, is also considered to be a sense-consciousness. But mental phenomena are also ideas, notions, and thoughts, not just sensations. Mindfulness is a true form of thinking, like free association in psychoanalysis. The second mode of perception is inference; it is discursive, speculative, and deductive. This mode of perception can also be correct or incorrect. When it is correct, thinking is aligned with the things-in-themselves. When it is incorrect, thinking is delusive or egocentric.

The Buddha may have been the first person to teach that ideas are just a habit of memory. Most of our ideas recall things in the past. However, this is a descriptive phenomenological observation. Ideas are habits of jouissance, and jouissance can be constructive or destructive. But ideas are also logical signifiers organized by language and culture.

## Samadhi Is a State of Non-perception

When sense-consciousnesses contact objects without the intervention of mind-consciousness, the world of suchness, the ultimate dimension can reveal itself. When mind-consciousness intervenes, however, it generalizes everything, and the self-mark of an object transforms into a universal mark of things in themselves into representations. The self-mark of an object means not that an object has a sense of self but that an object gives a sense of self to the subject. Our mind-consciousness tends to perceive the universal rather than the particular, relative, and egotistical mark of things.

Remember that the first seven consciousnesses—the sixth-sense consciousnesses of eye, ear, nose, tongue, body and mind and the seventh consciousness of *manas–vijnana*—all manifest from the eighth consciousnesses, or the store consciousness, which is unconscious and does not die, only evolve. This is part of the metapsychology or beyond psychology. The whole universe is a product of Mind rather than Mind being a product of material reality. This is definitely an idealistic conception of the universe as a product of the human mind, a form or creation out of nothingness or emptiness. Mind is not a product of material or social reality. Material reality is a product of unconscious Mind, in the big sense, not of the Freudian repressed unconscious.

Things do not arrive and depart. People either manifest or remain latent. If they manifest, they live in the world of karma or volitional action. It is unclear if latent thoughts or people produce any karmic results, although in Christianity, Jesus hardened the Jewish Law by saying it is sinful for a man to look at and fantasize about a woman twice, and vice versa. Desire may be a potentiality in our consciousness, but it may or may not manifest.

The school of Western psychology that primarily focuses on sensation and perception is Gestalt. It emphasizes how humans perceive objects as part of a whole system (inter-being and interdependence, in Mahayana Buddhism), rather than individual components, and has significantly contributed to the study of how we organize sensory information.

Cognitive psychology and behavioral psychology study mental processes and observable behavior through the senses. Mental process is not discerned as primary and secondary, as in Freud. Thinking and language in humans organize perception. Animals don't have language, only signs. Does this mean that they are in touch with the things-in-themselves and therefore are more Buddha than humans are? This would not be correct; therefore, thinking and language are necessary to reach a higher level of the things-in-themselves as emptiness.

When we open our eyes, what we see depends on, among other things, what is around us. But what is around us? Should we say that trees, furniture, and people are around us? Or should we say, rather, that what is around us are colors, shapes, sizes, and textures? Or should we perhaps say that what is around us are atoms, fields, and patterns of electromagnetic radiation? Even if reality is indeed made of particles, fields, and patterns of electromagnetic radiation, few of us would be inclined to say that this is what we see when we open our eyes. Physics teaches us that 'reality' is hidden from our senses, so whatever we see around us, be that trees and desks, or colors and shapes, these are only appearances.

In Aristotle's view, colors and shapes are real—as real as trees, desks, people, and other objects that are members of a totality that can be called 'reality' or 'the universe'. However, reality is not exhausted by material objects that can be seen, heard, smelled, tasted, or touched, for Aristotle thought that there are also immaterial objects, objects that cannot be known by perception but only by a special cognitive capacity that he called 'intellect'.

Aristotle agrees with his teacher Plato on many things about the intellect and its role in scientific knowledge (episteme), but he disagrees crucially about the role of perception. Plato thought that true understanding comes not from the senses but from recollection and rigorous dialectical exercises, which are often impeded by sense perception. Aristotle, by contrast, thought that true understanding must start with the senses. Freud and Jung are more allied with Plato, and behaviorism with Aristotle.

In *De Anima* 2.6, Aristotle (1956) draws a distinction between three kinds of objects of perception (or sensibles). There are two kinds of objects that are perceived directly, or in themselves, and one kind that is perceived only indirectly, or accidentally. Notice that he makes the distinction between in-themselves, or indirectly, and mentions accidentally rather than by images, as in Buddhism. What does this mean?

According to Aristotle, reality is organized by four causes and two accidental or chance forms of causality: automaton, which looks like an accident but had unconscious causes, and Tyche, a benevolent surprise or accident cause by our past good actions plus the unconditioned.

In England, Berkeley's idealism opposed Locke's realism, in that Berkeley believed that the physical world doesn't exist independently of the mind and ideas, while Locke believed that ideas are based in sensation and material reality.

Buddhism distinguishes among different types of perception, some false and deluded, and some true and enlightened. 'Delusion' does not mean a Western psychotic phenomenon but simply all undisciplined thinking. Thinking as well is distinguished as deluded and distorted thinking and correct and incorrect thought. Right thought is one of the limbs of the eightfold noble path to enlightenment.

For Freud, there was no concept of the things in themselves or of ultimate reality as part of the healing process of psychoanalysis. Lacan, however, had a concept of Thing and nothing as the things in themselves. Reality instead was given by language and visual perception. For Jung, however, visual perception was perception in images, which for him were superior and more symbolic than language. This would contradict both Buddhism and Freud. For

Freud, images were part of the primitive instinctual primary process and not ultimate reality, which was what Jung believed.

For Jung, archetypes presented themselves in disturbing and irrational images. They were not rational and were disturbing. The things in themselves are never disturbing; only perceiving them through images is.

## References

Aristotle. (1956). *Aristóteles: De Anima*. Edited by W. D. Ross. Oxford: Clarendon Press. The edition major, with an English introduction and a modest commentary by Ross, appeared in 1961 from Oxford University Press.

Freud, S. (1915). Metapsychological Papers. Collected Psychological Papers, Book IV. London: Hogarth Press.

Jung, C. G. (1961). Memories, Dreams, Reflections. Translated by R. Winston and C. Winston. New York: Vintage Books.

Jung, C. G. (2009). The Red Book. New York: Norton and Norton.

Susuki, D. T. (1960). Zen Buddhism and Psychoanalysis. New York: Harper Books.

Suzuki, S. (1970). Zen Mind, Beginner's Mind: Informal Talks on Zen Meditation and Practice. New York: Weatherhill.

Thich, N. H. (2001). Transformation at the Base: Fifty Verses on the Nature of Consciousness. Berkeley, CA: Parallax Press.

# 7 Teaching Psychoanalysis

Lacan cannot conceive what the future of his knowledge and his teaching will be, or the future of psychoanalysis. He (Lacan, 2005) talks about his teaching not being a pill or a form of medicine you can take to feel better. He ponders how his work will be remembered in future textbooks, and whether he will be summarized and dismissed in only three lines. In his book *My Teaching* (Lacan, 2005), he says that he likes a well-constructed dissertation with a start, a beginning, and an end, contrary to how he wrote the *Ecrits*, which were not systematic and which most people, even he, considered unreadable.

Everyone thinks they know what psychoanalysis is except for psychoanalysts; they're the only ones not to know because they have to not know in order to function as psychoanalysts.

Is sexuality central to what I teach or my analytic practice? Sexuality is in fact important to people, but other people in treatment complain about other things, not about sexuality, or have aspirations or value in life other than sex. Most people complain of not being loved enough by their mother, but failure in a good enough mother is misinterpreted as a rejection. Yet most maternal rejections are necessary Oedipal rejections signifying their allegiance to the Name of the Father (NoF.).

What do I teach about sexuality—a healthy genital life, like Freud desired, or the equivocation of sexual difference and desire? A healthy genital life leads to sex therapy and eroticism. What I teach about love and sex is Lacanian but with a twist. In Lacanian theory, love 'ex-sists' in RSI: the Real, the Symbolic, and the Imaginary. There is imaginary, symbolic, and real love. Real love is not reality love but empty love, where you love in the other what you love in yourself and love in yourself what you love in the other. So, in emptiness there is universal compassion, contrary to what Freud believed.

Lacan believed that there was no use in trying to make human society better like social theories, sociologists, and the Frankfurt School of critical theory tried to do. For Lacan, human society has always been madness and is none the worse for that. Society has always been madness and will always be like that. Having studied the Frankfurt School, I don't think I agree with Lacan. History does show signs of progress or a periodic return to the sacred origins.

DOI: 10.4324/9781003658702-7

Why do I speak of teaching in this autobiographical way? Well, I am one of few published Lacanian psychoanalysts in America. I think most people know me as also being a Zen teacher. There are not many psychoanalysts publishing in the English world anymore; many have died. However, there are many psychoanalysts practicing in America today, both inside and outside the American Psychological Association.

I have been interested in spiritual and intellectual knowledge since my adolescence. Once I graduated, I became interested in teaching, and I taught psychology until I, with several others, began a Lacanian school in San Francisco. Several of my publications helped make this a reality. Consequently, I started an online school in China. I teach knowledge of Freud and Lacan, psychoanalytic knowledge outside these two, and a psychoanalysis with Chan characteristics.

Lacan said that his followers called themselves Lacanians, but as far he was concerned, he was Freudian. It is true that Lacan studied Freud's work in great detail, more than other analysts of his time, but he focused his study in a particular way that in the end led him to develop his own theory of psychoanalysis and the unconscious in relationship to language and beyond.

I have studied Freud and Lacan following Lacan, but I have developed my own way of reading, studying, and interpreting Lacan's work. I have no interest in adding my name to the plethora of theories in the field of psychology. I would like to be remembered as an analyst and a writer, but not as the founder of a theory of psychoanalysis, but as a living psychoanalyst and interpreter of Lacan.

Obviously, there are many good translators and interpreters of Lacan's work, as there should be. My work differs in that I have studied and written about Lacan's seminars but have also added new concepts to develop the theory and the practice, following Lacan himself. Most people follow the Lacan of the middle period, based in his study and analysis of Freud's pivotal works. The later Lacan changed his view of the Real, which I capitalize, and construed the Real as jouissance and a new topological circle and knot that makes 'accord' or harmonizes. This introduces an element of holism that many will reject if they know about it. This moves away from Freud's dualism and the divided or split subject of the early Lacan. Not surprisingly, Lacan was interested in Chan Buddhism, as I covered in my book on Lacan and Chan (Moncayo, 2023).

My own way of reading, studying, and interpreting Lacan's work was not as a lone ranger singing "I did it my way". My professional practice and livelihood led me in this direction. I became a licensed psychologist in Berkeley, California, a degree that was needed to see patients and be a practicing clinician and professor. At this time, I wrote *Evolving Lacanian Perspectives for Clinical Psychoanalysis* (Moncayo, 2008). Lacan's approach to the clinical frame, standard and nonstandard, helped me apply psychoanalysis to outpatient psychotherapy in a public clinic.

In this book I worked on the problem of narcissism, classifying it into four kinds, normal and pathological. I also introduced the problem of sexuation and sexual difference, as well as the difference between biological and anatomical difference and sexual difference in the culture as man or woman. Some males identify with women and some females identify with men. In this book I also explored the *objet a* as the agalma or jewel in the Real.

I began my studies of psychoanalysis thanks to a fortuitous occasion. I was interested in Western psychology, but I was also attracted to Eastern spirituality without being a Jungian. I met somebody in Paris, France, who introduced me to Soto Zen practice, which I pursued after I came to California. Paris was also the place of Lacan's teaching, and he mentioned Zen in *Seminars I* and *X*.

To explore this twofold interest, I wrote *The Signifier Pointing at the Moon* (Moncayo, 2012), on psychoanalysis and Zen Buddhism. I begin by examining the cultural context for the relationship between psychoanalysis and spirituality. Psychoanalysis is a secular and nontheistic study of the Mind, the same thing that scholars say about Zen. In the West and in Descartes, meditation means thinking, while in the East meditation is not-thinking or trying not to think. Dōgen, in Japan, carried this further and spoke of 'non-thinking' instead of 'not-thinking', which he viewed as suppressing thought and the intellect.

Freud distinguished between the conscious and unconscious ego, Jung distinguished the Self from the ego, and Lacan distinguished between the ego and the subject of the signifier in relationship to language. I used this time to distinguish between conditioned consciousness and unconditioned awareness, both in Zen and in Freud's work (the mystical writing pad).

In response to multiculturalism in the clinic and the profession, I wrote *The Emptiness of Oedipus* (Moncayo, 2012). Rather than ego identity, as in ego psychology and object relations, Lacan spoke of the subject as a unary trace, nothing that could be easily championed as an ego identity. The unary trace comes from the Real, while on the basis of the trace, the ego identifies with traits of the Other/other.

Now, when I was licensed in California, I became acutely aware of the model of science that the APA uses for psychology. Psychoanalysis was also losing its scientific standing. I wrote the book *The Real Jouissance with Uncountable Numbers* (Moncayo & Romanovicz, 2015) with Magdalena Romanovicz, who was a brilliant intuitive mathematician. Lacan focused on the relationship between language and mathematics in his approach to science. In his *Seminar XIV*, he looked at the relationship between the capital Phi and the minus phi within golden numbers. Here is where I realized that these imaginary numbers had to be understood within the complex plane rather than the Cartesian plane, as the rest of psychological research does.

In my book on *Seminar XXIII* (Moncayo, 2017), I distinguish between the early use of the real and Lacan's later use of the concept of the Real. This also led me to distinguish between different types of jouissance. There are three basic jouissances: the jouissance of the Other, phallic jouissance, and the Other jouissance. The third jouissance subdivides into feminine jouissance, the jouissance of the mystic, and the jouissance of enigmatic reading.

My next two books were very important for my intellectual development. In my book on knowing and not-knowing within psychoanalysis (Moncayo, 2018), I address the similarities and differences between Pierce's theory of the sign and Lacan's theory of the signifier. I also clarify two different forms of probability and chance in Aristotle. Automaton, also known as 'fate', is compulsive and overdetermined, like the concept of karma in Buddhism. Destiny, in contrast, is undetermined surprising and beneficial. In my next book, *The Practice of Lacanian Psychoanalysis* (Moncayo, 2021), I distinguish between a DSM-5 approach to diagnosis and a Freudian anthropological approach to diagnosis. I also distinguish between the signifying chain and normative narratives in psychotherapy, as seen in the Lacan's graph of desire.

In my next book, on Lacan and Chan Buddhism (Moncayo & Yu, 2022), I zeroed in on the relationship between Lacan's Borromean knot and Vasubandhu's three-foil knot in Zen from the third century CE. I start by reviewing what Lacan wrote about Zen in *Seminar X*. I come to a new understanding of Freud's use of the Nirvana principle, since he only used the Hinayana or Theravada view of it. I also explored the different views of animal nature, human nature, and Buddha nature.

In *Lacan, Jouissance, and the Social Sciences* (Moncayo, 2023), I explored Freud's use of Darwin's concept of the primal father to document the history of culture and the economy. I examined the concept of labor in Hegel and Marx. Hegel has a view of alienated labor as necessary. Marx invented the concept of surplus value, which Lacan used to talk about jouissance and surplus jouissance. Marx did not think that people enjoy work that much, and he did not see how capitalists are rich because they enjoy their work, not only because they exploit the workers. In China, due to traditional meritocracy, workers enjoy work and thus became rich. Finally, in this book I discussed how jouissance and motivation work as the 'animal spirits' of the economy.

In my next book, on literature and psychoanalysis (Moncayo, 2024), I explored how Freud and Lacan thought that more could be obtained from literary books than from science for psychoanalytic practice. Modern English replaced religion for the general population and the world. Lacan's analysis of literature is based on his analysis of the letter as a unit of the signifier. But the letter is more than the signifier, in contrast to Derrida, who criticized Lacan for 'phallologocentrism'. Lacan considers literature (as fiction) as containing truths and logical fantasies. And of course Freud followed Jakobson in considering the Freudian mechanisms of condensation and displacement as synonymous with the formation of metaphor and condensation.

In a book on Lacan's *Seminar XX: The Torus of Reason* (Moncayo, Belnap, & Farr, 2024), I and my coauthors explored the question of the language of the One and the language of the Other to explain the differences between linguistics and the use of linguistics in psychoanalysis. The book is focused on a further exploration of Lacan's formulas of sexuation that I began in a chapter of my first book.

Finally, in the book *The Concept of the Individual in Psychoanalysis* (Moncayo, 2025a), I focus on how different theoreticians have conceived of the individual, culminating with Lacan's ego or subject of the Real. The latter is a form of jouissance, rather than an imaginary ego or a symbolic subject.

Following my book *The Real Jouissance of Uncountable Numbers*, focused on Lacan's *Seminar XIV*, my most recent book, *The Mind of Complex Numbers and the Subject in Analysis* (Moncayo, 2025b), is an attempt to develop a mathematical methodology to measure the effectiveness of psychoanalysis as a treatment. With a simple Likert scale, I measure symptoms before and after treatment. Then for each case I develop a list of key signifiers that appeared in the analysis with a corresponding reduction in symptomatology. Finally, I associate the capacity for sublimation that leads a subject to become 'weller' rather than well.

Finally, I wrote this, *The Knowing of the Psychoanalyst*. Here I think of non-thinking and truth as a state, and of the use of language to speak of the ineffable—discourses without words, which are not the master's discourse, but rather the silence of the analyst.

## References


Lacan, J. (2005). My Teaching. New York: Verso, 2008.

Moncayo, R. (2008). Evolving Lacanian Perspectives for Psychoanalysis. London: Karnac.

Moncayo, R. (2012). The Emptiness of Oedipus: Identification and Non-identification in Psychoanalysis. London: Routledge.

Moncayo, R. (2012). The Signifier Pointing at the Moon. London: Routledge.

Moncayo, R. (2017). Language, Sinthome, Lalangue, and Nomination: A Companion and Commentary on Lacan's *Seminar XXIII* on the *Sinthome*. London: Karnac.

Moncayo, R. (2018). Knowing, Not-Knowing, and Jouissance: Levels, Symbols, and Codes of Experience in Psychoanalysis. London: Palgrave and MacMillan.

Moncayo, R. (2021). The Practice of Lacanian Psychoanalysis: Theories and Principles. London: Routledge.

Moncayo, R. (2023). Lacan and Chan Buddhist Thought: Reflections on Buddhism in Lacan's Seminar X and Beyond. London: Routledge.

Moncayo, R. (2023). Lacan, Jouissance, and the Social Sciences: The One and the Many. London: Routledge.

Moncayo, R. (2024). Lacanian Psychoanalysis and American Literature: Metaphoric Truth, Imaginary Fiction, Letter Jouissance, and Nomination. London: Routledge.

Moncayo, R. (2025a). The Concept of the Individual in Psychoanalysis: The Ego, The Self, The Subject, and the Person. London: Routledge.

Moncayo, R. (2025b). The Mind of Complex Numbers and the Subject in Analysis. London: Routledge.

Moncayo, R., Belnap, B., & Farr, G. (2024). Exploring Lacan's Seminar Encore Seminar XX: The Torus of Reason. London: Routledge.

Moncayo, R., & Romanowicz, M. (2015). The Real Jouissance of Uncountable Numbers: The Philosophy of Science in Lacanian Psychoanalysis. London: Karnac.

Moncayo, R., & Yu, Y. (2022). Lacan and Chan Buddhist Thought: Reflections on Buddhism in Lacan's Seminar X and Beyond. London: Routledge.

# Index